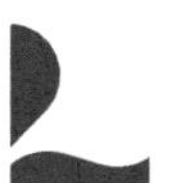

I0815529

TIM BOUTS

Diary of a Zoo Vet

Lannoo

Introduction

My parents had absolutely no special connection with animals. We had a dog and some chickens, but that was it. I am the youngest of three boys, the baby of the family. Stef was the oldest, then came Rob, and I came seven years later. As a child, I mostly looked up to my oldest brother Stef. He was a member of the pony club in Bocholt, and I loved nothing more than going along with him. In the summer, Stef and I went to the Geerits farm almost every day. Stef cycled while I sat on the bike handlebars, legs dangling over the front wheel. I spent a large part of my childhood on that farm; it was a great time, the so-called 'good old days'. When we joined the farmer for dinner, we drank milk straight from the cooling tank and had soup followed by potatoes from the same plate. No fuss, just the basics. We helped with various chores, such as milking, cleaning the stables and feeding the animals, before playing and riding the ponies. My pony was a Shetland pony named Kirsten, and this was also my first pony in the pony club. I was barely five years old, but I was already hooked. When I outgrew Kirsten, I continued with Kitty, Elske, and then Merrie.

I had a carefree childhood, surrounded by animals and friends. At home, I steadily expanded the number of animals: I bred dwarf hamsters, gerbils and chinchillas. I also had my pet rooster, Guust, who followed me everywhere. To the great despair of the neighbors. Ever since I was eight years old, I knew for certain: I'm going to be a veterinarian. I never considered any other profession since then. 'What if it's too much for you?' asked my father. He preferred that I go to Maritime College, something he would have liked to have done himself when he was young.

But not put off at all, I replied:

'We'll just wait and see. There's no other option.'

I started studying veterinary medicine in Ghent in 1994 and fortunately passed that first year. In my final year, I had to choose between treating cattle, industrial animals such as pigs and chickens, horses, or small pets. I chose cattle, believing that this would prepare me for working with large wild animals, which had always been my ultimate goal.

Especially because of my father, who had lived and worked in the Middle East for years, I developed a passion for traveling. I got to spend two and a half months in Vietnam for my thesis on parasitology. That trip to Vietnam was my first trip outside of Europe and my first experience with solo travel, a huge adventure that initially came with a massive culture shock. I lived with the locals, was part of their daily life, worked with them and spent time with their families. It was enormously enriching. However overwhelming that experience was initially, it turned out to be one of the most memorable experiences of my life. I can still remember the smells, the hustle and bustle, and the people in Vietnam.

When I graduated, I started my career in the Surgery and Anesthesiology department for large animals in Ghent, specializing in anesthesia. I already knew that I wanted to become a zoo veterinarian, for which anesthesia was very important.

I continued my zoo veterinarian studies in London at the Royal Veterinary College and London Zoo, where I followed an intensive training program for a year.

During that training, I started to grow as a veterinarian and eventually became one of the first Belgians to specialize in caring for zoo animals. I had the opportunity to work on various research projects and deepen my knowledge.

I traveled from London to many other cities, so gradually the whole world became my workplace.

I went to Abu Dhabi to investigate the deaths of hundreds of gazelles, to Whipsnade Zoo in England where I feared for my life during an attack by a chimpanzee, I met the Spix's Macaw at Al Wabra Wildlife Preservation in Qatar, the most endangered species of parrot that I would with others help to save from extinction, and I tried to resuscitate a baby orangutan at the Pairi Daiza Zoo in Belgium. These are just some memories off the top of my head, because with twenty years of experience, it's difficult to choose which stories have stuck with me the most. What's more, I am not only a zoo veterinarian, but have also worked as a zoological director for the past twelve years. During this time, I have learned that managing a zoo is much the same as managing people. Although interpersonal relationships are quite different from interacting with animals, I can say that I have managed like a veterinarian: there is a problem, a diagnosis, and a solution. That approach may be too pragmatic for some, but it certainly worked for me.

And above all, there is also my own story, that of my family, my wife and three children who are my world. Marie has been following me since day one, Jonah was one month old when he moved to Abu Dhabi, Jef was born two years later at the beginning of the Whipsnade period, and Laura-Marie was born in England three years later.

In a way, Kirsten the Shetland pony brought me from the farm in Bocholt to the whole world, from a little boy to zoo veterinarian. It has been an exciting ride, and along the way I have learned a lot and have been able to carry out various projects. Looking back on that journey, I know that this passion for animals has always been inside me. It is my calling and life's work to care for all those beautiful creatures and contribute to their well-being.

Meanwhile, I also know that being a veterinarian is more than just taking care of animals. It's more complicated than that. There is population management, research, conservation, and difficult decisions that need to be made when an animal escapes, as well as the ethical question of whether to carry out euthanasia. Furthermore, a zoo is more than just a collection of animals. It's a whole machinery, a concept. It's a world in itself, which tells the story of nature.

2002-2004: Belgium and Cornwall, England

After my studies in London, I temporarily returned to the Faculty of Veterinary Medicine in Ghent. I alternated this with weekend work at a veterinary practice run by friends: partly in Limburg where I'm from, and partly in Picardy in France. Meanwhile, I was so fascinated by wild animals that I was constantly looking for opportunities to work with them. One day I found the perfect job offer in Newquay in Cornwall: a mixed practice that was also responsible for Newquay Zoo, a small zoo which also had some interesting animal species such as fossas and kinkajous.

I took Marie with me for a weekend to have a look around, and we both immediately fell in love with Cornwall's beautiful countryside. On top of a cliff at Polly Joke Beach, with only a wild seal in the Atlantic Ocean below us as witness, I got down on one knee and asked Marie to marry me. Fortunately, she said 'yes', but not before I had to assure her ten times that I wasn't joking. When we got back home from that weekend, I had not only a new job, but also a fiancé. We got married soon afterwards and moved to our new home the day after our wedding, a place eleven hours away by car and boat from Belgium, deep in the Southwest of England.

The time we spent in Cornwall was wonderful. As newlyweds, we were lucky enough to spend our honeymoon in one of the most beautiful places on earth. We went for walks along the cliffs by the coast almost daily, just the two of us and our dog Bongo, named after a percussion instrument and an antelope. Bongo's name was settled pretty quickly, what with Marie's background as a musician and mine as a veterinarian. On a professional level, I learned a lot in Cornwall. It was my first experience with small pets like dogs and cats, but I also got my first zoo experiences at Newquay Zoo.

1. Suzy

The car's engine is roaring as I am busy with some maps. I try to flatten them on my thighs to get a view of my location, but there is not much space between the steering wheel and my upper body. The only thing I see are the green patches on the map, showing me the French fields I am lost in. I ended up here because I am gaining practical experience on weekends at a West Flemish veterinarian who has been living and working in France for over twenty years, in Saint-Quentin, a city in northern Picardy, halfway between Paris, Lille and Brussels. If I'm not working in Bocholt at another veterinarian's office, I spend the weekend here and have a room above the practice. The work I can do here is a great addition to my specialization in anesthesia and allows me to earn some extra money, because that specialization doesn't pay that much.

At the moment, I am expected by Jacques, a French farmer who has requested help for a sick calf.

I angrily throw the maps on the passenger seat and continue driving blindly. After a while, I approach the farm where I need to be. Jacques is already waiting for me.

'You know what breed it is?' he asks.

'The Blonde d'Aquitaine?' I guess. Belgium is proud of the Belgian Blue, while in France it's the Blonde d'Aquitaine. They are beautiful, elegant cattle, with fine skin and horns.

'They are known for their excellent meat,' I add, trying to be jovial.

'And their aggressive nature,' the farmer winks.

He leads me to the stables and I notice that the farm doesn't look very modern, to say the very least. It all comes across as a bit dirty and grimy.

We come to a dark stable, the size of a kitchen, with straw and thick metal bars you have to work your way through to enter.

'There lies the calf.' Jacques nods towards a corner of the barn, while the mother cow is peacefully ruminating in the other corner.

The calf lies there, motionless. I enter the stable, kneel down next to the calf, and lift its head up. I think I can't possibly save this animal. But I have to and want to try.

I review the differential diagnosis: young calf, three days old, severe diarrhea: E. coli, rotavirus or coronavirus, cryptosporidium or coccidia. This differential diagnosis is drilled into you at university. Given the age, E. coli is the most likely, as the viruses occur around nine to ten days old, cryptosporidium around two weeks, and coccidia usually in calves of a few months. This is not conclusive, but I still decide to start a treatment for E. coli.

I pinch a fold of skin in the neck. It just stays upright instead of springing back flat. I open the calf's mouth and push my finger on the pink gums turning them white, then count: '1...2...3...4...5...6'. Normally, it should take no more than three seconds for the white gums to turn pink again, but here it takes twice as long. This calf is extremely dehydrated. The ears and mouth also feel cold, and the thermometer reads 92°F, so hypothermic, too. I need to administer a warm intravenous infusion of antibiotics and then subcutaneous fluid as well. I find the jugular vein with some effort, then insert a catheter. I connect the fluid and start the therapy.

All the while, the calf lies still without reacting.

I explain to the farmer, 'I'll come back tomorrow. Give me an update on how things are going. Especially if things don't go well, so I don't have to make the whole trip for nothing...'

I expect to quickly receive a phone call with bad news, but it doesn't come. I hear nothing from Jacques. The next day I drive back through the French fields, this time without getting lost, and look for the calf. Hopefully it's still alive.

'Fantastic!' Jacques calls out to me as I arrive. 'I don't know what you did, but that calf is back on its feet!'

Jacques's enthusiasm may be a bit exaggerated, but the calf has indeed made progress. It stands up straight again and reacts alertly to our presence. The mother also looks at us curiously.

'Wow,' I say immediately. I hadn't notice yesterday how impressive the mother is, even with her horns sawed off.

'That's Suzy,' Jacques nods. 'One of my best and most beautiful cows.' He leads me into the stable to do my work, but when I grab the calf, it gets scared. It starts mooing towards its mother, upon which the enormous cow turns towards me and charges without hesitation. Before I can respond, she headbutts me and pushes me over. I fall to the ground with a hard thud.
I hear the farmer curse while I see him fleeing from the corner of my eye through the thick bars.
'God damn it,' I think.

With my arms in front of my face and upper body, I quickly try to get back up.
But Suzy gives me another headbutt.
And another. She keeps pounding me, right on my chest, and I can't move.

I'm terrified and try to protect myself from this violence, but don't think I'll make it out alive. I get more and more scared with every blow, and the seconds feel like hours... Please let it be over soon.
'I'm coming!' I suddenly hear the farmer shout. He races back into the barn with a thick metal rod in his hand.
'Allez!' he bellows while hitting Suzy with the rod. It works. Suzy gets distracted and takes a few steps back, allowing me to finally escape. On hands and knees, I crawl through the bars. My whole body hurts. I drop myself on my back as soon as I'm safe and then lose consciousness.
'Tim? Tim, are you okay?'
I open my eyes and am somewhat reassured that it's Jacques hovering above me and no longer Suzy. I immediately feel the pain in my body again. My sternum and ribs are in bad shape.
'You've been lucky,' says Jacques. He can't hide his own relief. 'Suzy is my most aggressive cow. Those horns weren't sawn off for nothing...'
I shake my head and try to get up.

'That calf still needs to be treated...' I groan.
'Not until I move Suzy,' Jacques says dryly.
A little later, I lower myself gingerly onto the car seat. I want to sigh, but even that hurts. Everything hurts. Instead of driving straight to the vet, I stop by the hospital. I undergo the necessary examinations and receive the verdict: no broken ribs and no collapsed lung. Bruising and a lot of pain, though. But especially the idea that this job involves more risks than I previously thought. As a young, recently graduated veterinarian, you're fearless and think you can take on the whole world, but an incident like this brings you back down to earth. Suddenly you're mortal and realize that one wrong move can turn your whole life upside down.
When I return to the vet's office late that night, he looks at me in surprise.
'Where have you been?'
'Underneath Suzy,' I groan, grimacing
'Suzy!' he laughs. 'I know her. The most dangerous cow in the area!'

2. I am not a doctor

'He's having trouble breathing.' The elderly lady sounds concerned as she places her parrot's cage on the examination table in the practice in the Cornish town of Newquay. I can tell her husband shares her concern as he nods in agreement. The lady carefully takes the parrot out of the cage. The man gives him a little kiss on his beak. This animal is loved, that much is clear.
Jeff, the parrot, looks around curiously, but I indeed hear its labored breathing. Many people don't realize it, but the examination of the sick animal begins when the owner walks in with it. Every step and every bit of information is a piece of the puzzle that I, as a veterinarian, try to put together in search of what is wrong with the animal. And what the solution could be.
'Let's take a look,' I say reassuringly.
As always, I start with an anamnesis on which I then base my differential diagnosis. That's a kind of standard questioning of the owners I use to learn more about the animal, its housing, diet, and the problem. I already know the problem in this case, but how long has it been going on? Has the parrot been sick or treated before? How is its eating and drinking behavior? Does it eat a lot of sunflower seeds? The more precise the owners answer those questions, the better we can determine where the problem might lie.
I then look at things like the animal's posture, condition and behavior before moving on to a general examination. In this case, I focus on the breathing, paying attention to its frequency, type, and rhythm. I also check for the presence of white plaques in the parrot's nostrils. Such plaques occur in Hypovitaminosis A, a disease that occurs when birds are fed exclusively seed mixtures, especially sunflower seeds. I check for the presence of white spots in the mouth, something we often observe in cases of parasitic or fungal infection.
'The nose and mouth look good,' I say after that check. Meanwhile, I'm thinking of psittacosis, also known as parrot fever. The disease

is caused by the bacterium Chlamydophilla psittaci. After infection, there is often a reduced appetite, dehydration, diarrhea, and inflammation of the eye and nasal mucous membranes, which can lead to respiratory problems as in this parrot. If diagnosed early, the disease can be effectively treated with antibiotics.
'I'm going to take a quick swab of the mucous membranes,' I explain. The lady and gentleman nod in agreement. As long as it benefits their Jeff in the end.
'I think it could be chlamydia. It's very difficult for the little guy now, but with an antibiotic treatment we can make him better.'
I send the couple home with Jeff and a prescription for doxycycline, telling them to come back if there's no improvement. A few days later I receive confirmation from the lab that my suspicion was correct: the parrot tested strongly positive for chlamydia. I give the owners a call to assure them we started the correct treatment. The lady answers the phone. She sounds tired.
'Doctor...' she says, which usually makes me laugh because I am not a doctor, at least not a medical doctor. But I hear her voice break. 'Jeff is better, but my husband... He has been admitted to hospital with severe lung problems.' They think he has cancer, but for now they can't find anything...'
While the lady tells her story, my gears start turning. The man is having trouble breathing and they can't find anything. During their consultation, I saw him giving kisses to the parrot. The parrot has chlamydia, which is a zoonosis, an infectious disease that can be transmitted from animals to humans. People with a weaker immune system are more susceptible to infectious diseases in general, but this also applies to zoonoses. This risk group is summarized in literature as 'YOPI': Young, Old, Pregnant, Immunosuppressed which means young children, the elderly, pregnant women, and immunocompromised individuals.
'Ma'am...' I ask cautiously. 'May I call your husband's treating physician with your permission? I might be able to help...'
A little later I speak to the doctor on the phone.
'If I may...' I say cautiously. 'The man's parrot is undergoing treat-

ment for chlamydia, and it may be a possible avenue to also test the man for this zoonosis. The issues can then be resolved with antibiotic therapy.'

'You may...' I hear the doctor say. 'But if I may: you have no authority as a veterinarian. I examine and treat my patients, people, in the best possible way. So a veterinarian shouldn't be telling me how to do that. Thank you for your call, Dr. Bouts. Goodbye.'

Surprised and a little angry, I hang up the phone. Although the reaction of that doctor is over the top, it does illustrate the difference between a veterinarian and a human doctor. A veterinarian constantly thinks in terms of trans-species, as we are accustomed to looking at different animal species. We simply consider humans as a species of animal, albeit perhaps the most foolish of the primates. Humans and animals can never be considered completely separate from each other, as proven by transmissible diseases. When a disease passes from animal to human, we want to know how that happens. Does it transmit through breathing, excrement, objects, or are there other possibilities? In a zoonosis, we try to establish a first barrier to infection: disinfecting hands, wearing gloves and face masks, avoiding contact, and so on. In that sense, veterinarians are to some degree responsible for protecting society, hence the checks on the import of animals or at slaughterhouses. It would only take one mishap for the world to be turned upside down quickly.

I have no regrets about my phone call; I wouldn't be doing my job properly if I hadn't informed the doctor of the facts and my suspicions. It's just unfortunate that he didn't want to hear it and considers his own status more important than his patient.

I let it go, and a few weeks later I see that Jeff the parrot has a scheduled appointment.

The elderly couple enter the consultation room with a smile.

'And?' I ask curiously. I knew the parrot would be alright, but the husband...

'Jeff seems perfectly healthy again,' the lady says.

'And I feel the same way,' the man laughs.

His expression says it all.

'I really wasn't doing well, but at a some point the doctors switched to a different treatment and I fully recovered.'
'Thank you, doctor,' says the lady.
Then it's my turn to smile. 'I'm not a doctor, you know.'

3. DIY

'I have a little job for you,' says my boss. 'A wild sparrow hawk has just been brought in.'

He nods his head towards the examination room. I have only been working in this practice for four weeks, so I'm pleased my boss already has so much faith in me.

I nod confidently and enter the examination room.

They found him in Weybridge, in the open fields not far from the coast, says Sheila, the head nurse of the practice. She carefully opens the box on the examination table, which contains the sparrow hawk. 'He definitely flew into something. A power cable maybe, or a window. His right wing is drooping and he can no longer fly.'

'Hm,' I say. 'Hopefully no broken wing then. We'll take a look.'

It's a beautiful creature, its feathers shining in grayish hues. I presume it's a male, as they are often smaller than females. The bird is clearly flustered when we look at him. He looks up and has his talons ready to defend himself if necessary. I carefully reach into the box to grab the bird by its talons. In a bird of prey, those talons are actually the most dangerous, not the beak. He flaps around wildly with one wing, while the other hangs limp next to his body. I touch and look at the wing, and it's immediately clear that something is indeed wrong with it. There's an open wound and the humerus, the upper arm bone, is sticking out. An X-ray needs to be taken to confirm exactly what kind of fracture we're dealing with: is it simple or are there multiple fragments, and how far is the fracture from the joints?

'That'll be anesthesia then?' says Sheila, who immediately springs into action, preparing everything. Sheila has at least thirty years of experience as a nurse, which always puts me at ease, although she may not realize it.

I nod. We anesthetize the sparrow with a small gas mask and then insert a tube into its trachea. We position the wing of the bird on the radiography cassette to get a good view of the fracture.

On the X-ray, it's clear we are dealing with a simple fracture. The fracture is in a good location, not too close to the shoulder joint, but will need orthopedic treatment.

'Have you ever done something like this before?' Sheila asks.
I hope she isn't asking that question because I'm getting nervous. Because I have never done 'something like this' before.

'I've only had a class where we had to break a bone in a dead pigeon and put it back together.'
'It's almost the same thing,' Sheila laughs. The fact that she's on board should reassure me.
Because it won't be easy. Sheila needs some time to gather all the materials, as we will be using what looks like homemade crafting material.
'Here you go,' she says proudly, arriving with a tray containing all we need: pins, various sizes of injection needles, infusion tubing and a special two-component hoof glue called 'technovit'.
Now we can get started.
'Take your time,' Sheila says, before I can muster up the courage myself.
Because courage is what I need.
Birds have hollow bones, so they are light and can fly effortlessly. When one of those bones breaks, you can mend it by sliding a pin through the bone to reconnect the two parts of the fracture line. When you do this, the two fracture halves can still rotate relative to each other. So to fully stabilize the fracture, a kind of stabilizing bridge is made to hold the bottom and top of the bone in place.
I try to stay as calm and composed as possible while following the steps in my mind. My hands are not shaking, I notice. I control my

breathing and take my time.
I feel like a real handyman,' I remark halfway through the operation. 'A DIY enthusiast working on a PROJECT.' Sheila laughs, understanding what I mean.
The X-ray after the surgery shows that my handiwork is perfectly in place.
'Good?' Sheila confirms.
'Very good.' I feel proud.
To finish it off, I cross the two tips of the wings over each other on the back and stick them together with a piece of tape, so the bird can't spread them.
'Did it work?' Sheila asks as I drop my hands next to my body and tilt my head slightly toward the bird, as if admiring my handiwork.
'It worked,' I confirm.
It was my first surgery on a bird of prey, and a wild one at that, so I'm glad everything went well. Now I can only hope that he recovers well. The sparrow hawk stays with us in the practice for three weeks and kind of becomes my buddy. Every day I check on him and the wing, which seems to be healing well. Several weeks pass and the X-rays confirm that everything is fine. I can now remove the pins and needles. The bird moves its wing a little more every day, until it can fully open and flap with it again. Now it's time to move him to the Cornish Bird of Prey Centre for further rehabilitation. If all goes well, he will be released back into the wild.
A few weeks later, my boss calls me in again.
'The sparrow hawk,' he says. 'Do you still remember that bird?'
I nod and wait anxiously. Has something gone wrong?
'Congratulations,' he continues. 'You did a good job.'
I try to keep my *cool* while beaming with pride.
'The bird can be released back into the wild. The people from the rehabilitation center called asking if you want to be there. That might be fun?'
'For sure!' I reply enthusiastically.
The next day I'm standing on the plain where the sparrow hawk had been found injured, together with two colleagues. This place is so in-

credibly impressive. For me, it may well be one of the most beautiful places in the world. I see fields and rolling hills as far as my eyes can see. And way out in the distance I can see the coast. It's very windy and cold, but the sun warms me up. I have to squint my eyes to see into the distance.

'Are you ready?' I hear.

With a big smile, I nod.

'I'm ready.'

The door of the kennel is opened and then turned away from us.

With my camera in my hand I am ready to capture this moment I never want to forget.

The sparrow hawk cautiously steps out of the kennel. He looks around curiously, spreads his wings, and then... flies away.

We silently watch the bird as it eventually disappears as a small dot on the horizon.

For the first time in my life, I was able to release a bird back into the wild. What an incredible, powerful and beautiful feeling.

2004-2006: Abu Dhabi

When I was studying in London, I had the opportunity to go to Peru for my Master's thesis to work with small South American camels, vicunas. Geer, a nature lover through and through, had arranged this for me. A few years later, when I was working in Cornwall, he called me asking if I wanted to come work in Abu Dhabi for the private wildlife collection of the Crown Prince of the United Arab Emirates. Marie was pregnant with Jonah at the time and we were happy with our life in Cornwall, but curiosity led us to a weekend trip to Abu Dhabi. The project that was presented to me was incredible. It was a nature conservation project aimed at protecting mainly antelopes and wild goats, the Arabian tahr goat.

Marie and I decided to go to Abu Dhabi together, but first we would enjoy the birth of our first son, Jonah, in Belgium. When he was one month old, I left for Abu Dhabi alone. Marie and Jonah followed a month later. The reunion with my family was wonderful; I had missed my wife and son terribly.

The project became a major challenge, both professionally and personally. The collection of animals was spread out over six different zones and every day I had to be somewhere else. I traveled long hours and mainly treated large groups of animals in vast areas, but also took the time to care for individual animals when necessary. Especially with the Arabian tahr, of which there were only about fifty individuals left in the wild, each animal was important. For this species, we set up a breeding program and were able to save them from extinction. Friday was my day off, and then I was expected at my Emirati boss's private zoo. A small but fantastic zoo, specialized in breeding cheetahs and other rare felines. Even though this was work, Marie and Jonah almost always joined me and we always made it a fun day. When hand-rearing the baby cheetahs, Marie gave them a bottle while Jonah played with the kittens in the nest.

The Arabic culture was completely new to us and we were a little worried about how it would be for Marie as a woman. However, this fear turned out to be completely unfounded, as all people, including the Emiratis, were extremely friendly. A blue-eyed blond baby naturally helped every time we were introduced. Jonah often went from arm to arm among young and old, men and women. The biggest downside was the absence of our families who lived more than 4,000 miles away, but that was compensated by the close friendships we developed there. At the end of the day, every expat was in the same boat as us.

We mainly spent our free time in the countryside. After a twenty-minute drive, we could go swimming, just across the border in Oman, in the wadis that had nice cold water all year round with waterfalls. And this was the desert! We often camped with our friends Grant and Angie, both animal managers, at Abu Al Abyad along the beach, and then had a nice South African barbecue, a 'braai' as they would call it.

In the United Arab Emirates, I have learned in particular to distinguish between the importance of the group and the individual animal when it comes to my job as a veterinarian. The approach is completely different in both cases, but one is not more important than the other. I have also learned a lot on a personal level. We worked for and with billionaires and people of different nationalities, religions, cultures, and backgrounds. Tolerance, patience and above all respect were key every day in working together and achieving some wonderful things.

4. That's my job

Grant and Angie are waiting for me at their dwelling: a square block with air conditioners on the wall, in the middle of the desert. They wave enthusiastically as I drive into the compound, but all three of us know that the reunion is not just for pleasure. On the contrary. Grant and Angie are animal managers who asked me to drive out from my house in Al Ain, which is inland by the Oman border, to Abu Al Abyad. That's roughly 155 miles away, on the coast between Abu Dhabi and the border of Saudi Arabia. Home to 40,000 antelope, Abu Al Abyad is the second largest antelope reserve in Abu Dhabi, and probably also in the rest of the Middle East. The animals live in the wild on an island in the Arabian Gulf, but are under the supervision of Grant, Angie, and their team of keepers. The phone call I received from them this morning was disturbing. They had found 50 gazelles dead. That may seem like a negligible number out of a total of 40,000, but when sudden mortality occurs in a population, there is usually something more going on. And I'm here to figure out what.

I park my car in a shaded spot and quickly grab my backpack from the passenger seat. I gathered some things before I left, assuming that this job wouldn't last more than a day.

'Smart,' Angie says, pointing to the backpack. 'I'm afraid we have a serious problem on our hands.'

We don't want to waste any time, so Grant and Angie immediately take me to the place where the carcasses are located. They had collected these this morning during their feeding round, after which the resident veterinarian already performed some autopsies.

In a clearing shaded by a few palm trees, the carcasses are piled up on top of one another. It is as impressive as it is unsettling.

'Not good, eh?' remarks the resident veterinarian.

I shake my head.

Updating me, he explains:

'We found all these animals dead this morning, scattered across the

island. The keepers contacted me and I immediately asked them to collect the carcasses and bring them here. Meanwhile, I called Grant to come here as well, so we could look at the animals together. I have examined some of them and they all have similar symptoms that are limited to the chest cavity. I've never seen this before, and don't know what to make of it. Hopefully you know more about this. I'm at my wits' end.'
He sounds desperate and I am eager to start the post-mortem examinations.

I drop to my knees next to one of the lifeless gazelles, and even though I've seen these animals up close before, it's overwhelming. Such graceful animals aren't meant to lie dead in front of me, let alone in such a heap.

I take my scalpel, prepare some jars with formalin for further histopathological examination, and some swabs for bacterial examinations. I briefly hover my surgical knife above the skin I'm about to cut into. Begin.
When I open the chest cavity, I shake my head.
'What's this...' I mutter in surprise. My colleagues, Grant and Angie, are looking over my shoulder. 'I've never seen this before. Hepatization of the lung...'
Hepatization is a change in lung tissue, making it resemble liver tissue. There are also fibrin strands hanging against the lungs and chest cavity, which is filled with a bloody fluid. I look up and glance at the other gazelles. This cannot be a coincidence, and, as contradictory as it may sound, it's good that there is not just one dead animal but that I can also examine those other gazelles. After several autopsies, it appears that, as my colleague had already suggested, each gazelle exhibits the exact same symptoms.
In the evening, I retreat to the guest room at Grant and Angie's

house to do some research. I need to know where this is coming from and, in particular, how we can prevent it.

'Tim?' Angie gently knocks on the door and cautiously sticks her head through the doorway. 'Don't you think you should come and eat something?'

I nod. To stay sharp, I also need to take care of myself. I follow Angie outside, where it has finally cooled down a bit. Grant is sitting at a lavishly set table, staring ahead. I slide onto the seat next to him.

'It's so unreal,' he says, shaking his head. 'We have been bush guides for so long and worked with wild animals all our lives. We know them inside out. Every slightest change in their behavior, gaze, demeanor... nothing escapes us. These wild animals are our whole life. But as soon as it becomes medical, we don't know what to do. It feels like the animals are slipping through our fingers and we are powerless. We simply don't know what to do.'

Angie lowers her head in sorrow, her eyes glistening. A large group mortality of the gazelles would be a disaster. In the Arab world, religion is very important and according to that religion, animals should not be sick. Because of their long history as nomads, animals are considered a status symbol here. Keeping falcons, sheep, and goats symbolized wealth in the past, but today they've been replaced by gazelles and cheetahs. The nomadic lifestyle has ended, but the love for animals remains. Every disease outbreak is therefore a disaster for various reasons.

'You don't have to do anything,' I reply. 'That's my job. And I will do my best.' If I don't owe it to the animals, I certainly owe it to Grant and Angie, two gems of people.

Instead of going to sleep after eating, I continue doing my homework. My head is spinning with thoughts and emotions: how could this have happened? What do I tell the boss? How can I help Grant and Angie? What is this damn disease? Until I suddenly find it: contagious caprine pleuropneumonia or 'CCPP'. That's a disease that occurs in goats in Africa and Asia, and is caused by Mycoplasma, a bacterium. The germ causes a severe infection of the lungs, with morbidity rates reaching up to 100 percent and mortality rates of up to

80 percent. The symptoms are completely consistent with what I read in the literature, but of course we need to have it confirmed by the lab. If it's this, it will be disastrous. And that's confirmed the next day. Together with Grant and Angie, I drive through the gazelles' habitat. Angie speaks first: 'There.' I look to where her finger is pointing and see a dead gazelle lying a few meters away.
'And there,' Grant adds, bringing the car to a stop.
'There,' I also say.
During our drive, we end up finding 80 dead gazelles. It's terrible. We all have tears in our eyes.
Upon returning to the compound, we brief the team.
'It's a battlefield,' Grant says quietly. 'Every animal needs to be rounded up and removed. I'm sorry,' he concludes. He wants to apologize to his team, maybe even to the antelopes themselves. But there is nothing he could have done about this.
I start with the autopsies and there is no doubt about it: all these animals died as a result of CCPP. This is then also confirmed by the lab.
The next day we are back in the jeep. Grant, Angie, me... No one says a word, we are too afraid of what we will find. Not 50, not 80, but 120 twenty dead gazelles.
Angie breaks the silence as we drive back.
'I'm devastated...'
I can only nod in agreement. Even though it's not my fault the animals are getting sick, I still feel responsible. They're all counting on me to do something, to stop all those deaths. It weighs heavily on me, but I certainly mustn't show it.
The mortality is spreading extremely fast and needs to be brought under control. I need to try to contain the outbreak, or better still, try to stop it on an island of 184 miles2 with all its roaming animals, but for now that can only be done through trial and error.
Since the bacterium is inside the cell, it is difficult to treat with antibiotics, as most antibiotics cannot penetrate the cell. This means we have to wait for the bacterium to come out of the cell to infect another cell in order to kill it. Moreover, gazelles are ruminants and can't receive antibiotics orally, as it can ruin the entire rumen flora.

That's what we are taught at university. However, this is the only possible way because of the size of the population and the environment: how can we treat that population efficiently?
So keeping in mind the principle of 'damned if you do and damned if you don't', I try to administer an antibiotic treatment through the feed. I start with a safe broad-spectrum antibiotic that can be administered orally in other, non-ruminant animal species. The gazelles are fed every day during their regular feeding rounds, so it's just a matter of adding the antibiotic to their feed.
'This won't be easy,' I say during a team meeting. 'The only way to administer the antibiotics is by mixing it with their feed. The 55-pound bags of pellet feed that you already use will need to be mixed with the antibiotic.'
I see someone frowning, probably because they are wondering how on earth we're going to do that.
'With cement mixers,' I explain. 'We will reduce the amounts of food to make sure everything is eaten and they receive the antibiotic.'
The frowning gives way to nodding; everyone is on board.
'It's the first time ruminants are being administered an oral antibiotic on such a large scale,' I conclude. 'We'll have to pull out all the stops.'
The team is not lacking in motivation, so everyone immediately springs into action.
The team starts with food preparations early in the morning and is only finished with the feedings for the next day at night. Everyone works nonstop, willing to do anything to treat the animals.
'It's not working,' says Grant after two days. He sounds defeated, but doesn't want his team to hear so as not to demotivate them.
'They keep dying,' he says. It's what I was afraid of.
Because the mortality rate is not decreasing, I realize I need to try something else. I change strategy and use a different type of antibiotic used in chickens with Mycoplasma. The mortality rate decreases, but not quickly enough.
'We are still losing too many animals at too high a rate,' Grant informs me again.
'Okay,' I say immediately. 'I'm going to take a risk, okay?' I say.

I want to give a combination of two antibiotics. It has a very bitter taste, so the pellets will need to be mixed with oil and powdered sugar to remove the bitterness.

'Do you have time for a trip to the grocery store?' I ask. On the way there, I explain my strategy to Grant.

'So we're going to buy powdered sugar?' he summarizes.

'A lot of powdered sugar.'

The man in the supermarket looks surprised when we buy all the powdered sugar in the entire country. Another three days later, I am once again sitting in the passenger seat of Grant's jeep early in the morning. The sun casts a beautiful glow over the island and the sea. I lower my binoculars for a moment and close my eyes, the sun burning my face.

'This is good,' I hear Grant say, more to himself than to me.

We don't come across a single dead gazelle throughout the entire journey. The mortality rate really has decreased. We have won. The gazelles have won. Once again we have tears in our eyes, but this time from joy.

It ultimately takes three weeks to complete the treatment. But it doesn't stop there. With CCPP, there are three possibilities from the moment you treat an animal. Either the animal dies, the animal gets better and the bacteria disappears, or the animal becomes a carrier of the bacteria. The last option is the most dangerous, because in that case the disease can come back. To prevent that, all the animals must be vaccinated. And that's difficult, as the gazelles live in the wild here. But difficult works too! Temporary mobile shelters are built where we feed, capture, and vaccinate the animals. It's a huge task that takes several months, but after that the disease never came back. Twenty years later, I am still friends with Grant and Angie, and every time we see or hear from each other, we talk about this story. We are still proud of what we accomplished together back then. It's cases like these that form real, close friendships.

5. Close the curtains

The powerful sound of the spinning rotor blades above my head is impressive and drowns out everything else. The helicopter hovers hundreds of meters above the ground, allowing me to enjoy a panoramic view of the landscape below us. I'm in a military helicopter being escorted from my hometown in Al Ain, on the border with Oman, via Abu Dhabi to the island of Sir Bani Yas. It's a one-hour flight instead of a three-and-a-half-hour car ride. On the island, which is the United Arab Emirates' recently deceased president's private property, the animals have been able to breed for years without any form of maintenance or conservation. As a result, the animal population is bursting at the seams and I have been asked to look into what can be done about it.

The helicopter maneuvers smoothly and I get yet another unique perspective of the surroundings. It's fantastic.

'Have you been able to spot a dugong or manatee yet?' The pilot looks at me with a smile, as he speaks into his microphone. I shake 'no' with my head, with my headphones on. The dugong is one of the animal species I would love to see in the wild. My eyes once again scan the water bordering the desert, but no manatees in sight. I do see several antelopes and giraffes, like miniature versions of themselves due to our great height. While landing, I put away my hopes until the return flight and focus on the reason why I am here.

'Mr. Bouts, welcome!' a man shouts enthusiastically at me as I step off the helicopter. It's Mike, the supervisor of the island. He immediately takes me to his jeep to show me the island.

'I'm curious,' I say.

'You'll be amazed,' he enthuses.

We are not even five minutes into the drive and I already feel like I'm in Africa. We pass animals everywhere. The miniature giraffes and antelopes I saw from the air now take on realistic, impressive proportions. There are many of them. A lot. Really a lot.

'Where do we start...' I mutter, somewhat impressed.
'The total capacity of the island is around 25,000 animals,' Mike explains. 'But there are easily twice as many here.'
I gulp. 50,000 animals? In this area? That's mission impossible.
'There's a lot of uncontrolled growth,' Mike continues. I've only been here for a short while and know I'm here for precisely that reason, but it still surprises me to see it in real life.
'We'll sort that out,' I say firmly, trying to convince myself as well.
I review the information I need to resolve this overpopulation. How big is the island? How many animals are there? What animals are there? How many males are needed for the females? In the case of gazelles and antelopes, for example, only one male is needed for every five to ten females. So counting will be necessary. And the animals need to be caught so that the males and females can be separated. In total, about 25,000 animals will have to be relocated to other nearby breeding centers.
'We need help,' I declare to Mike as I explain my plan. We neither have the manpower nor the resources to carry out such a large operation. That's why I am enlisting the help of South African 'game catchers', specialists in catching animals on this enormous scale. All the necessary material will be shipped by sea from South Africa to Sir Bani Yas. The transportation takes several months, but when I receive word back in Al Ain that the cargo has arrived, I make sure I come not long after. I say goodbye to Marie and Jonah for a few weeks. They will be staying in Al Ain, as it is not ideal for them to join me in Sir Bani Yas.
During the helicopter flight to the island, I try once more to spot a manatee, but I quickly get distracted by what I see on the ground in the distance. It looks like a carnival being set up, what with so much equipment being dragged around and assembled.
'Mr. Bouts, welcome!' Mike says again when we see each other. 'It's incredible.' His eyes widen as he gives a huge smile.
Like a small child showing off a new toy, he takes me to where the animals will be captured to be then separated and relocated. The system being used is actually quite simple. First there is a wide, large

area the animals will be led into. The area covers several square miles and continues into a kind of funnel, preventing the animals from turning around. This becomes narrower and narrower until there is just enough room to let a number of animals through. To manage the influx, various areas are closed off every 54 to 109 yards with curtains that have metal joints from top to bottom, preventing the animals from escaping. At the end of the system, the curtains are replaced by metal panels, allowing all the animals to be sorted and vaccinated individually. Males and females are classified separately: either the animal stays on the island, or it goes to a facility to be moved later.
The first day I participate in the trapping, I am nervous. This is a huge operation that depends on the cooperation of everyone involved. Through my headphones, I hear the rangers' briefing in the desert. They're chasing the animals with their jeeps towards our trap system, which goes into effect immediately.
'They're coming!' I hear. In the background I can hear the sound of the jeep as well as the trampling of the animals. I'm standing on the side of one of those huge curtains and have to wait for the signal to close it. Someone will meet me on the other side with another curtain, so the space is closed off once those curtains touch.
It's extremely hot, the sun is burning, and I feel the sweat dripping down my back. I can't afford to make any mistakes. No one can, otherwise the whole system stops working. I prick up my ears and try to hear when the animals are coming, until the rumbling suddenly gets very close. I barely dare to blink as hundreds of gazelles rush past me through the funnel. The deafening noise seems to rise from the dust floating above the trampled ground.
'Close the curtains!' I hear through my headphones, so I immediately start to run. With all my strength, I pull the curtain behind me until I reach my colleague who is doing the same from the other side.
'Fuck', I say, even though I know I'm not supposed to swear. What's going on? The gazelles are futilely butting against the curtains on the other side. I don't know what I hear, see, or feel. This is so impressive...
Each day we do this all over again and let ourselves almost get literally trampled by hundreds, even thousands of animals. I spend

most of my time vaccinating the animals. I stand on a platform from which I inject the animals at the end of the funnel.

With my sweaty hands, I hold a 'polestick' all day long: a long stick with a needle used to administer the vaccines for rinderpest, foot-and-mouth disease, contagious caprine pleuropneumonia that has already caused mass mortality in one of the other centers I am responsible for, and Clostridium.

'Done!' I call out when each group has received four vaccines. The partition wall then disappears for a moment, after which the group of animals is reduced further. The males go straight ahead to a truck that transports them to another enclosure or off the island, while the females are led to the right where they are released back onto the island after the whole procedure.

It takes three weeks to get the entire island in order and bring the animal population to acceptable levels. For three weeks, about 50,000 animals pass through our hands, so to speak, and end up where they need to be. And it was kept that way.

Not much later, the island became a popular holiday destination where you can go on safari. A trip that I, in small part, have helped to make possible.

2006-2011: Whipsnade Zoo, England

After working in Abu Dhabi for two years, I started to feel the urge to be closer to home again. The absence of our families started to weigh on us, and Marie was meanwhile pregnant with our second son, Jef. I saw the job offer for veterinarian at Whipsnade Zoo in England, the sister zoo of London Zoo. I applied and, to my great joy, got offered the job.

We packed our things and moved to England. The first few months we didn't have a house and camped in various colleagues' houses, Marie, Jonah and I. Marie and Jonah eventually went to Belgium for a few weeks to prepare for Jef's birth, and I arrived just in time to witness it.

My boss Andrew, one of the most fantastic people I have ever met, was married to a Thai woman. He told me the following at the time: 'Tim, entire families live together in Thailand. My wife would be angry if I didn't ask you to come live with us until you find a house.

And so Marie, Jonah, baby Jef, and I set off back to England, to temporarily move in with my boss. Eventually, we found our home about 3 miles from the zoo in Dunstable and after some fixing up, we moved with our family to our first own little house.

At work, I became more and more integrated, and loved every second I was there.

The species of animals captured my imagination: elephants, rhinos, both white and Asian, giraffes, tigers, lions, bears, and more. It was one big amusement park for me.

Elephants quickly became my absolute favorite, and I spent a lot of time in the elephant stable with the keepers. We researched the ultrasound anatomy of the elephant eye and the radiographic anatomy of the elephant's lower leg. Unfortunately, we also had to deal with some deaths due to the elephant herpes virus, which prompted us to start researching this dreadful disease.

My other great love remained anesthesia, and with eight hundred wallabies and four hundred Chinese water deer living semi-wild in the zoo, I had more than enough opportunities to develop new anesthesia techniques. I also developed a protocol to calm large wild animals, just enough so that they would remain upright so we could still perform all the examinations we wanted. This was the most wonderful time of my career in veterinary medicine, and I will never forget the tremendous kindness of the people we met there. Also the delightful British sense of humor.

Here, we welcomed to the family, after two fantastic sons, our equally fantastic daughter, Laura Marie. We called her the snow baby, because Dunstable was completely snowed under when we had to rush to the hospital for the delivery. With the arrival of Laura-Marie, our family was finally complete. Marie regularly played in various orchestras and gave music lessons, and we had fantastic friends. The little brothers were already going to school and spoke better English than Dutch. They grew up, and Marie and I grew along with them in so many ways.

6. Pointing fingers

I have a healthy dose of nerves on my first day at Whipsnade Zoo. It will take some time to get to know the animals, but my colleagues are also new to me. I am to work with a team of nurses here and will also gradually get to know the keepers. Those are usually pleasant encounters and the contacts I have with everyone are always valuable. For example, I never question zoo keepers. These people know their animals the best, so if they say something is wrong with an animal you better take them seriously.

'It's incomprehensible,' says Julia softly. She's standing next to me in the specially equipped autopsy room at the zoo. She's one of the regular keepers of the kudu lying dead in front of us.

'He was perfectly healthy, nothing wrong.'

'We'll take a look,' I say quietly. I want to treat both Julia as a keeper and the antelope itself with respect. I carefully open up the antelope to perform an autopsy, looking for a possible cause of the sudden death. I'm focusing on the lower abdominal region, as the animal underwent a vasectomy three days ago for contraceptive purposes. It would be unlikely, but perhaps something went wrong there?

I open the threads of the surgical incision, spread the skin open with a wound retractor, and expose the surgical site. Then I hesitate. Surprised, I take a closer look.

'What's wrong?' Julia asks immediately.

I want to be sure before I give her an answer, so I double-check if what I see is correct: my colleague who performed the vasectomy tied off the urethra instead of the vas deferens. That's a serious mistake. A fatal mistake, even.

By ligating that urethra, the bladder could no longer be emptied and the urine flowed back to the kidney poisoning it. That proved fatal for the animal.

'Do you see this?' I ask Julia. 'This is the urethra. It should normally have a free flow, but that's not the case here.' I point with my finger.

'Oh no...' Julia shakes her head disappointedly as she works through in her mind what happened.

'So... this is due to human error?' she asks, even though she knows the answer.

I nod. 'I'm afraid so.'

'Oh no.' She puts her hand in front of her mouth. 'John... He definitely didn't do this on purpose... Will he get in trouble?'

'I do have to report this', I say almost apologetically, but Julia immediately nods.

'I have to take pictures of everything we see now, and I'll write down everything as accurately as possible so that I have all the facts when making the report. Facts that cannot be disputed.'

'Of course, sure,' Julia nods. She understands, but is distraught. I would also prefer not to do this, but I have to.

When I write the autopsy report a little later, I repeat to myself: I have to report this. And that's annoying, because I don't want to get my colleague John, whom I haven't even met yet, into trouble. He made a mistake and that's simply human. It is a challenging region to operate in, there are many blood vessels. Maybe he had a bad day or was distracted. It could happen to me too, so I don't want to publicly shame him, nor point fingers at him. I am even inclined to defend him... But still, the result remains the same. He simply should not have made that mistake, as it caused an animal to die. This could cost him his job... And I'm the one leading him towards that possible dismissal. I need to inform my boss, and I want to speak to John in person and inform the other keepers. I sigh. This is far from a nice first introduction to the team.

I attach my report in an email and send it to my boss, who doesn't immediately respond.

A day later, I receive a phone call. On the other end of the line is John.

'I apologize...' he says immediately. 'I have to make this phone call from my boss, but I wanted to call you myself anyway.'
'I appreciate that, John.' This must be a very difficult phone call for him, so I don't want to make it even harder for him.
'I shouldn't have made that mistake... But it happened. I wanted to quickly handle that vasectomy before your arrival and I botched it. There's nothing more I can say. I feel really bad about it.'
I know now that he is a resident physician, which means he is still in training. He shouldn't have even performed that procedure without supervision anyway. But I'm not going to blame him for that as well. He's probably already aware of that, and I suspect he has already received a full reprimand from the boss.
It's exceptional for something to go wrong during such a routine operation. The two procedures that a veterinarian in the zoo performs most often are castrations and vasectomies, which are always done as part of contraception. Whether it's the first or the second procedure depends on various factors. Not least how the animal or its environment responds to it, because castration of a male animal can change the whole dynamic in the group. For example, a lion would lose its mane after castration, and castration is never allowed in deer. The antlers are hormonally controlled in deer, so when a deer is castrated and the testicles are removed as a source of testosterone, the antlers will no longer fall off but continue to grow. In that case, a 'wig antler' develops, which can grow to an enormous size over time. So such actions must always be taken in the best interest of the animal. And most importantly: the correct procedure must always be followed, whether it concerns a castration or a vasectomy. 'To err is human', I say finally. 'And we just have to learn from our mistakes.'
And how is John doing now? Well, John has learned from his mistakes. He works well with the other colleagues and no longer performs surgeries that require supervision. He remains motivated, but combines this motivation with collaboration.

7. Near miss

Coco doesn't immediately throw poop at me, so she doesn't seem to be too bothered by my presence at the moment. From behind the bars of her enclosure, we look each other in the eyes. She looks at me defiantly; she knows that my arrival rarely brings good news for her. Chimpanzees are highly intelligent animals; they remember who they think is good for them and who is not. Who anesthetizes them against their will, for example. And so does Coco. Coco is a well-known chimpanzee who lived in London Zoo for many years before moving to Whipsnade. She's very recognizable to the public, who always calls her by her name. Furthermore, Coco is much smarter than the other chimpanzees and constantly observes the keepers and learns from them. I try to pass by her and the other chimpanzees as little as possible because they recognize me immediately and start to feel stressed; their adrenaline rises and when I have to sedate them, that adrenaline blocks some of the anesthesia receptors. This not only complicates the anesthesia, but also the further examination. Today, I have to perform a heart examination on Coco with a team of human doctors. So it's important that everything runs smoothly.

The examination is part of a heart program at the sports university, where we put all chimpanzees under anesthesia to examine their hearts. The 'Big Ape Heart Project' has been rolled out across Europe and we are the first ones putting it on the map. Great apes are getting increasingly older and also develop heart diseases with age. When a young chimpanzee suddenly died, the autopsy revealed that he suffered from a heart disease that also occurs in humans as a familial genetic disease. That is a huge source of information for us. The more we know about those great ape's hearts, the more we also learn about the similarities with the human heart, especially the heart of an athlete.

The chimpanzees here have been trained by their regular keeper Kathy and two animal nurses to receive injections by hand, to the

extent that they simply offer their shoulder on command and can be injected. Before the injection is given, Coco receives Valium. That way, she reacts less quickly to the injection, so we have a greater chance of success. It also blocks short-term memory so Coco won't remember she got an injection from her favorite keeper. But Coco clearly isn't in the mood for it today. She stubbornly refuses to eat the Valium and forces us to try another way.
'Yogurt it is then,' I suggest to Kathy. Kathy immediately starts working with the nurses; they know the protocol. A container of yogurt is opened, the Valium is added and Coco is lured again. But when she curiously accepts the jar through the bars, I see her hesitate.
'She knows.' I shake my head. She realizes the jar has already been opened, while she would normally open it herself. Plenty of reason for her not to trust the whole thing.
We try again, unsuccessfully, after which I switch to a different tactic. I suggest fruit juice. And then we try lemonade. But Coco keeps stubbornly refusing.
I review my options. If something goes wrong during a procedure, it often happens right at the beginning. Like now. Wouldn't it be better to stop then, I wonder.
'Okay', I finally decide. 'Let's carry on, but without Valium.'
Kathy nods. We both know that it's not ideal, but Coco has made it very clear in the past hour that we have no other option. I don't want to burden her with this stress and distrust again, hence my decision.
With a steady hand, I prepare a dart containing the sedative. I attach the dart to the gun. I have done this so many times that it seems routine, but you should never become nonchalant. Every animal is different and every anesthesia is different; that's something I am and will always be aware of.
Coco is sitting in a corner of her cage, and Kathy and I walk into the keepers corridor.
'Stay close to me,' Kathy says as we stop in front of Coco's enclosure.
I follow Kathy with the gun hidden behind my back. Coco must not become even more suspicious.
'Good girl, Coco,' I hear Kathy say. Coco immediately responds to

our presence in the keepers corridor and sits up. Over Kathy's shoulder, I see her positioning herself like a soccer goalkeeper: her back slightly bent, her arms outstretched, ready to intercept a possible tranquilizer dart in flight. Her posture and stature are imposing; she wants to intimidate us.

Kathy opens the fingers of her hand, as a sign that I should keep quiet and position the tranquilizer gun. We have to wait until she is completely still, and seize that moment.

And that moment arrives. Kathy clenches her fist, which is my signal to shoot. The dart hits Coco right in her side. But she quickly pulls it out and defiantly throws it down at my feet. I know the dart did hit her and I can see that it has fully discharged its contents; but to fully administer the medication, it needs to stay in place for a little longer than a second. So I am not certain because of her quick response.

'We have to wait,' I say softly to Kathy, who nods in agreement.

Coco retreats to her corner, and after a few minutes she starts showing signs that the anesthesia is starting to work. She visibly calms down, spins around dizzyingly, and eventually lets her large, cumbersome body sink to the ground. That is my signal to perform a check. It involves several steps. First I call out.

'Coco!' She doesn't respond. Then I clap my hands a few times, also without response, which proves that her auditory stimuli have disappeared. Then I poke her with a stick through the bars. Her response to objects has also dissipated.

Kathy and I give each other a nod. It worked, finally. Coco is out.

Kathy opens the door of the cage and since I have the responsibility as the veterinarian who administered the injection, I walk into the cage first to put a blindfold on Coco. After I'm done, my two nurses come in with Kathy and an additional keeper, in total silence.

Together with Kathy, I give Coco one final strong push to make sure all responses have been shut down. Meanwhile, the nurses are standing by with equipment to insert a tube into Coco's windpipe so the procedure can begin.

'Can I have it,' I say to one of them, signaling for her to hand me the tube.

But suddenly Coco opens her eyes. Two dark eyes immediately fill the room with fear. The nurse and I recoil, Coco jumps up and everyone scatters. With a sleepy growl, Coco prepares to attack and only has eyes for one person.

'Tim! 'Get out!' Kathy shouts. I feel Kathy pulling me back by my collar. The other keeper grabs my arm at the same time and helps Kathy to get me out of the cage as quickly as possible, with Coco's deafening roar behind us. I stumble and trip, running for my life until the door behind me slams shut.
'The nurses!' I say panicky as I sink to the ground, but Kathy shakes her head. 'They're okay', she puffs. And that's true. Coco has already calmed down, sitting in her cage slightly dazed, without even looking at the nurses.
'You. She just had to have you,' confirms the second keeper.
He lets himself fall against the wall just like Kathy, trying to grasp what just happened.
'She was faking it...' I say with a trembling voice. 'She acted as if she was sedated to take revenge.' No one had noticed. I didn't either, even though I know it can happen. She once again proved how intelligent she is. Though I don't think these theatrics were necessary.
I try to calm myself down, which isn't really working, because we can't stop here. Coco really needs to be sedated now, if only to check if she's okay after this stressful event.
I pick up my gun from the ground and prepare everything again, but now with a larger dose and a different anesthesia cocktail. My previously steady hand is now trembling. I'm shaking, and my breathing is fast and irregular.
'Will it work?' Kathy asks while she prepares herself for round two as well.

'It has to,' I say, mostly to encourage myself.

Just like before, I follow Kathy to the enclosure until we're close enough to Coco to shoot.

She assumes that goalkeeper stance one more. I feel overwhelmed by the sense of responsibility. This can't go wrong again. Kathy clenches her fist to say I can shoot now. I have to shoot. I hesitantly stretch my arm with the gun in my hand as I look at Coco. It's either her or me, that's how I feel. I shoot. I try to do it as quickly and as controlled as possible, but I feel like everything is happening in slow motion. The dart hits Coco in the shoulder this time, and she doesn't manage to pull it out of her skin quickly enough, because she thought it would be shot into her butt again.

Everyone anxiously counts down the seconds until Coco completely drifts away under anesthesia. I do the initial tests again. I call her name, clap my hands and poke her. No response.

I'm supposed to enter the enclosure now, but don't want to anymore. I'm just too afraid. Kathy and my nurses realize it too.

'Are you okay, Tim?' I want to nod, but I hesitate. I don't recognize myself. I'm distraught. Never before have I felt fear like this, never before has a procedure gone so wrong. This was my first *near miss*. And let it be my last. I know I have to enter the cage and do my job. I'm thinking of what parents say to their children when they fall off their bike: get back on that bike as soon as possible. And pedal. So I decide to pedal.

I gather all my courage and step back into the cage, blindfolding Coco and doing what I have to do with the help of the nurses. This time it works, but I don't feel at all comfortable.

When I write the report of Coco's procedure that evening, I wonder if I could have done anything differently. Or if I should have done something else. That question leads me to the Valium. I note that in the future no procedure should be performed without first administering Valium, as it blocks short-term memory, but also calms the animal slightly, resulting in somewhat slower reactions. Something we could have definitely used today. I also decide that ketamine should no longer be used for anesthetizing chimpanzees, but another narcotic, called zoletil, as in my second dart. Ketamine is known as a party drug in the nightlife scene, and Coco found that out today after her first dart, which was only partially injected. Zoletil is a combination of zolazepam and tiletamine and is a much stronger narcotic, causing the animal to go deeper under anesthesia even with a partial injection. Because of Coco, I am changing the protocol to be followed, so that no one else will ever end up in this situation again. I had a lot of respect for Coco and that remains the same, but she did stitch me up. Still now, I have an irrational fear of chimpanzees.

8. A not so sudden death

'Steffi is lying dead in the stable.' Steffi's keeper is upset when he tells me about it. Losing an animal is like losing a good friend for a dedicated keeper, and for some even like losing a child. So I understand where his emotions are coming from. Steffi is a giraffe that has been living in Whipsnade Zoo for years. It was a healthy and content animal, so its passing feels very sudden. Every animal that dies in the zoo must undergo a post-mortem examination, so that's what I'll do.

I stroke Steffi's fur when I sit with her. The fur feels normal, the animal looks okay, but she has lost weight recently. It looks like she's just sleeping.

Due to her sudden death, Steffi is labeled 'peracute mortality syndrome'. It is one of the leading causes of death in giraffes and indicates an unexpected death, seemingly without any apparent reason other than weight loss. The term 'peracute' or 'sudden' is actually considered incorrect, as the weight loss does indicate a chronic condition.

To examine Steffi, I first make an incision in the chest cavity and cut through the ribs with a heavy pair of pliers. The lungs and the heart appear normal at first glance. Then I open the abdominal cavity along its entire length, about 24 inches. After opening the abdomen, the intestines are exposed, and that's quite a lot in giraffes. Just like cows, they are ruminants and have four stomachs, actually three forestomachs and one true stomach, and a very long intestinal tract to digest leaves. When I open her abdomen, a kind of foamy substance flows out of the incision's opening. I take a sample of this liquid to determine the acidity of the rumen later. I dab the foam with a cloth, revealing that her rumen papillae are completely flattened. The papillae are supposed to be long and nicely rounded, so this is not good. This can only be the result of years of consuming the wrong food.

I check the rumen fluid with a test strip and, as I feared, I confirm that the acidity in the rumen is very low, 6, while it should be around

8. The balance is completely disrupted, indicating rumen acidosis. Due to this low acidity, digestion is disrupted and normal feed intake is adversely affected.
I realize that Steffi's death was not sudden. Her death was a slow one, and we weren't even aware of it. The reason: a nutritional issue. Unlike many of the large herbivores that alternate between leaves and grass, giraffes are almost exclusively browsers: they only eat leaves and the protein-rich shoots of trees and shrubs in the wild, and will never eat grass. The composition of leaves and grass is completely different, as leaves have a much higher protein and fiber content than grasses. The tropical world has no problem providing enough leaves, as there are always plenty of leaves available throughout the seasons. In Europe, however, that's not the case and there are only six months each year when fresh leaves can be found. Those other six months, therefore, we try to bridge with grass hay and sun-dried alfalfa hay, a roughage with high nutritional value due to the leaves that are included in the bale.

Our post-mortem findings confirm that the lack of leaves during half of the year puts Steffi and other giraffes in captivity in trouble. It is almost certainly also why giraffes are one of the few animals that live longer in the wild than in captivity.

I immediately realize that we need to fundamentally change how we keep giraffes in zoos in temperate climates like ours if we want to protect them from so-called peracute death. We can do that by drastically modifying their diet and better meeting their nutritional needs. This inspires us to establish a plantation of food trees in England that we can then prune in a rotation system to feed the giraffes. I also meet with our botanical department to coordinate tree pruning at the zoo with the zoology department, and involve volunteers to help preserve the leaves in the same way we store corn for our cows, to use as food during those difficult six months. We order large barrels to store the leaves in. During pruning, the smallest branches and leaves are pressed into the them. I jump into the barrels to pack the leaves as tightly as possible and we fill them all the way to the top, so that there is no air left before we put the lid on and store the barrels for our giraffes.

In captivity, animals cannot find their own food, so the responsibility lies with us. Spiders, mice, reptiles, felines, anteaters, elephants... The animals that live in a zoo are all so different. Some animals adapt easily to captivity, while others do not. This is often due to their diet. It's therefore extremely important that keepers realize the seriousness of all individual nutritional needs and the consequences if they are not met. Then things do go wrong. A simple and somewhat exaggerated example is this: a gorilla receives the perfect nutrition and follows a diet put together by the veterinarian: leaves, vegetables, and alfalfa pellets. He certainly won't get any fruit, because wild fruit has a different consistency than cultivated fruit. The keeper follows the plan perfectly, but let's say that one day that gorilla doesn't eat his cucumber. The cucumber is replaced by a banana with good intentions, and because the gorilla likes the banana, he will always be given a banana in the future. After that, he abandons the lettuce and it's replaced by caviar. And when the gorilla stops drinking water, he gets champagne. That's what we call 'nutritional keeper drift', and in this sense, keepers are the first *line of defense* in veterinary medicine. In itself, it's not really that strange that it happens. As mentioned earlier, the keepers regard their animals as their own children, and that's wonderful. But what a child wants is not always best for them.

'Is it my fault then?' Steffi's keeper asks when I share my findings with him. He knows what keeper drift is and I know for sure he would feel terrible if he were unconsciously guilty of it.

'Could I have done anything differently?'

'You didn't know there was a problem,' I reassure him. 'No. This is not your fault.'

9. Code red

'Code red! Coco and Phill have escaped! Code red!' I hear through the phone.
'I'm coming,' I say calmly, though suddenly I feel my heart pounding. I immediately hang up and hastily gather some things. My wife looks at me with concern. It's Sunday and that's a day of rest for us here in England. The children are still walking around in their pajamas, breakfast is still on the table.
'Code red,' I now say myself. Marie immediately knows what that means and says nothing more.
Every zoo has an escaped animal protocol, a kind of roadmap that tells you what to do when an animal escapes. Every two months, a zoo has to conduct an exercise, an escaped animal drill, where they run through that protocol.
It starts with giving a code. Code yellow means a harmless escape, for example a small monkey or a bird breaking out. Code orange is for animals that could be dangerous depending on the circumstances, such as medium-sized felines like servals, caracals, or large antelopes. In that case, we must try to sedate the animal as quickly as possible. Code red is when a dangerous animal has escaped like a lion, tiger, or chimpanzee. There is then a 'shoot-to-kill' policy: if necessary, the animal may be killed.
Thanks to the existing protocol and those drills, everyone normally knows what to do for each type of animal. Staff on site have to keep a safe distance from the animal and find a safe place to protect themselves; other staff need to evacuate to a safe location and stay there. An assigned staff member updates everyone who doesn't have access to walkie-talkies by phone and acts as an intermediary during the emergency. And the 'core team' consisting of the veterinarian, the zoological manager, and the marksmen prepares to immobilize the animal as quickly as possible. The veterinarian goes to the hospital, takes the tranquilizer gun, and prepares an anaesthetic dart. The zoo-

logical manager and the marksmen go to the 'armory' to get the guns and ammunition. When all this is done, we meet at a safe place close to the escaped animal to decide whether the animal can be anesthetized or needs to be euthanized.

While I'm on my way from home to the zoo, the entire protocol automatically kicks in. The zoo is still closed at this hour in the morning, so an evacuation of visitors is fortunately not necessary.

I'm trying to stay calm. I know it involves Coco and Phill, two adult chimpanzees who have been living in captivity for years. Coco lived through the days when chimpanzees were hand-reared, back in the 1970s. That was possible because these animals are extremely intelligent and also attached to humans because they were raised by them. The chimpanzees became so tame and accustomed to 'free contact' that in England they served as companions at tea parties organized by the nobility. Those were tea parties where the chimpanzees had to serve as entertainment, dressed in human clothes and provided with a table of food and drinks. Something that thankfully is no longer allowed today. Coco has already surprised me once by faking that I sedated her, and I feel a special vibe around her, as if she sometimes wonders why she's with all these weird animals instead of humans. And today she apparently took her chance to leave those animals...

When I arrive at the zoo hospital, I know no more about the escape than when I had left home.

I immediately grab my walkie-talkie and the first thing I hear is: 'Phill has been eliminated. I repeat. Phill has been eliminated.' One of the keepers then enters the hospital.

'Phill is dead,' he says. 'Trevor had to shoot him.' Shaking his head, he sinks down onto a chair. I sigh. Trevor is also one of Coco and Phil's regular keepers. This must be terrible for him.

'And Coco?' I ask immediately.

'Ron and Don are still working on that.' He shakes his head, which doesn't give me much hope.

Later that day, everyone sits dejectedly in the meeting room. A debriefing has to take place to determine what happened, where things initially went wrong, how quickly the response was, and so on.

The atmosphere is both tense and somber. Trevor looks as white as a sheet, Don stares into space, and Rob keeps shaking his head. Around 9:30 a.m., I reported the escape,' he explains. He speaks softly and slowly. 'It's my fault that Coco and Phill were able to escape. I forgot to close the doors when leaving the enclosure... I thought... I didn't know they were in their enclosure.'
Everyone is quiet as a mouse. Rob has been the keeper of the chimpanzees for years, he knows them inside and out. He would never act so recklessly, never make such a mistake. And yet it happened. He even didn't forget to close one door, but three doors. Three SAS doors that are meant to prevent such an oversight from leading to an escape. Rob had made a human error today. His first mistake ever, but one with disastrous consequences.

Trevor continues. 'Coco and Phill immediately ran to the top of the hill. Coco disappeared from my sight, but I had Phill within shooting distance. So I shot. His screaming seemed like... It was as if I had shot a person...'
The meeting room is quiet as a mouse.

'I jumped in the car with Don,' Rob continues a little later. 'Don was standing in the back of the pickup truck with his gun, while I drove around. I kept calling Coco's name until she emerged from the woods. I knew she was harmless at that moment, but Don remained on standby. Coco recognized me immediately, she opened the car door herself and sat on my lap. That confirmed my suspicion that she had assumed we were going to a *tea party*, like she used to... Don informed the team via walkie-talkie to open the doors of the outdoor enclosure so we could simply drive in.'
Rob hangs his head, he is clearly devastated. He also knows that Coco could just as easily have been shot if it had not been him, but

someone else in that car at that time. That's why it's so important that keepers also have a license and are part of the *gun team*. The keepers know their animals, they know when to shoot or not.
Both Rob and Trevor made the right assessment today, even though everything feels wrong.

10. Is euthanasia an option?

A transport box is being unloaded from the truck. There's no sound coming from the box. Though that's what you would expect, knowing it contains a pygmy hippopotamus. The box is loaded onto the truck using a forklift, so it can be transported to the indoor enclosure. Our new resident wakes up and starts shaking the box as it hangs in the air on the fork. So there's definitely a hippopotamus in there then. Ella has come from Portugal to Whipsnade Zoo as part of a breeding program. We have a male pygmy hippopotamus here, but we need a female to breed. And that will be Ella.

The box is placed in front of the gate of the indoor enclosure, and some food is placed inside the enclosure so Ella will be more inclined to leave her transport box. The large hatch of the box opens and we watch curiously as Ella hesitantly takes a few steps and slowly enters her new home.

The welcoming of a new animal is always a special moment, as if someone new is joining the family. But as romantic as that may sound and as fun as it would be to organize a family party, there is also a practical side to the story.

Ella hadn't been quarantined by the Portuguese zoo before this move. The British authorities therefore expect us to adhere to a mandatory quarantine period and test the animal for possible diseases. If we want to prevent diseases from spreading under the radar, quarantine and testing are actually the only ways to do that.

After a few days of acclimatization in her new home, it's time to sedate Ella for her tests. I shoot a dart just behind the ear, because the skin is thinnest there, and wait for her to fall asleep. I collect some blood samples from one of the rare superficial blood vessels in the foreleg and perform a tuberculosis test. Tuberculosis is a contagious disease that occurs worldwide, in both humans and animals, as it is a zoonosis, a disease that can be transmitted from animals to humans, and vice versa.

The chronic disease may develop years after infection, and transmission is possible through airborne spread, but also through milk, saliva, and feces.

To perform that tuberculosis test, I have to administer two injections, one with bovine and one with avian PPD. That's a purified protein derivative of either bovine or avian tuberculosis. We give both injections to distinguish between true tuberculosis (bovine tuberculosis) and false tuberculosis (avian tuberculosis). The injections are given at the base of the ear auricle, intradermally, meaning in the skin, so we can easily check for any swelling. The bovine PPD goes in the right ear and the avian PPD in the left. After three days, the test can be read: if the swelling on the bovine side is larger than on the avian side, then the test is positive. And what do you know? Three days later, I see that the skin in both auricles has reacted strongly to the injection, and it is clear that the right side is more swollen, so Ella is now officially suspected of TB.

That's reason enough for me to take a moment to think, because now the roller coaster will start. The possible infection has to be reported to the official government agencies, and Ella must remain in quarantine until we receive official confirmation from the government on the next steps. Things that all sound simpler than they are. A pygmy hippo is not like someone you can keep in their bedroom for a few days.

Once at the office, I call DEFRA, the Department for Environment, Food & Rural Affairs.

'We have received a dwarf hippopotamus from Portugal that has tested positive for TB.' I present the facts clearly, so that an accurate assessment can be made of the necessary next steps.

'Hm,' I hear the voice mumble on the other end of the line.

'I'm informing you so that we can intervene,' I explain further.

'Well, that test isn't recognized for pygmy hippos here,' he says. 'So for us, it doesn't really matter.'

I can't believe my ears. This can't not matter surely?

TB is such a contagious disease... If we were to release Ella in the zoo, the damage would be immeasurable.

During a meeting with the keepers, we discuss the situation.
'I think that we should take responsibility ourselves,' I suggest. 'If there's no protocol to follow, we'll create one ourselves.'
Everyone nods and realizes the risks Ella carries.
'What's your plan?' asks Tessa, one of the keepers, giving her trust in me.
'We'll draft it now, together.'
First and foremost, we need to be sure if it really is TB. I know I cannot retake the TB test right away, as there is a waiting period of 42 days. Moreover, I want to have some certainty quicker. I still have blood samples and manage to find a TB specialist who works at the Animal Health Agency in Weybridge. He can perform molecular tests on the blood to detect TB. I contact him right away and he suggests sending the blood samples for further analysis.
A few days later, I pick up the phone and call him.
'A bit of mixed news,' he says immediately when I have him on the line.
'The first rapid test gives strongly positive results, but the second, more specific test, a MAPIA (multi-antigen print immuno assay), cannot confirm this result for now.'
I nod.
'Ella is therefore suspected of TB but this is not yet conclusive,' is the verdict.
There is no other option but to wait out those 42 days and retest Ella herself with the PPD injections and a new blood analysis. A bronchoalveolar lavage (BAL) will also be performed. This is a technique where fluid is injected into the lungs and then aspirated back in the hope of collecting tuberculosis particles. After three days, the swelling in the outer ear is even more pronounced and the rapid test comes back positive again. The MAPIA test will also provide clarity this time. Antibodies are detected against the bacterium responsible

for bovine tuberculosis and against some specific antigens of this bacterium.
It must now be assumed that Ella does indeed have TB. She is a potential danger to other animals and people who come into contact with her. Especially as keepers, we also need to protect ourselves when handling her. Something that causes great concern for one of the keepers. It's Tessa, the keeper who first showed me that sign of trust during our meeting.
'I can no longer work with Ella,' she says one day. 'I'm sorry.'
She shakes her head apologetically, but I know what this is about. From the first suspicions of TB, Tessa had told me that she suffers from an autoimmune disease. If she were to become infected with TB, it could be fatal for her.
'You don't have to apologize,' I assure her. The others nod in agreement.
'I also think it's too dangerous,' says another keeper while raising his hand. I fully understand how they feel. These people work day and night with their animals, they would do anything for them. For Ella as well. But risking their own health is too dangerous; that's something no one can or should expect from them.
'Well, then maybe euthanasia is the best option in this case?' I cautiously suggest.
The decision to proceed with euthanasia is not one I make alone and is not taken lightly. The most important assessment we need to make in Ella's case is whether the risk of spreading the bacteria is manageable or not manageable. In other words, is it feasible to isolate her for a period of six months? That is the time needed for treatment. Because there is a treatment, although an expensive one. If we were to start that treatment, however, it would mean that we would have to keep Ella out of the water all that time. We would have to prevent any form of spread, including and perhaps especially through water. The water in her enclosure cannot be filtered, and it is discharged into a stream that runs through other animal enclosures. Furthermore, we cannot just keep Ella out of the water for six months. She is currently being sprayed enough, but as a semi-aquatic animal, she

needs more than that to ensure her well-being.
All those arguments are collected and laid out on the table during various meetings, with the keepers, the animal team and the management.
'So we have a decision,' we all finally conclude together. 'We will proceed with euthanasia.'
Tessa looks down, clearly struggling with this decision. No one in the room is having an easy time; I can tell by the despondent looks of the keepers and a sigh from the management. Still, we all stand behind our decision, as we made it as a team. Not only is euthanasia the best option for everyone's well-being in this case, it is also the best option for Ella herself. However contradictory that may seem to some, it is actually the most logical option.
Everything revolves around animal well-being, and reduced well-being stops with euthanasia.
A day later, it's time. I get the gun ready while my nurse Jo prepares the sedative dart.
With one shot, I hit Ella. The injection will work quickly, causing her to fall asleep. It takes a few minutes, but then Ella slowly sinks down to the ground. She finds a comfortable position and eventually falls asleep.
'Call the keepers,' I say to Jo. With euthanasia, it's customary that keepers who wish to do so can say a final goodbye to their animal. I step out of the box to give everyone privacy. Tessa is the last one to say goodbye to Ella. Her eyes are teary as she comes out of the box. I nod at her, she nods back. There are no more words to say. This is not what we wanted, but we know that it's the only option.
'Can I stay?' she asks.
'Of course.'
Together with Jo and Tessa, I enter the box again. I draw more blood for further tests and administer the injection for euthanasia into a blood vessel in her foreleg, so Ella's heart will stop beating and she can peacefully drift off. Everything is done so that the euthanasia proceeds correctly: painless, fast, simple, irreversible, safe for me as the person administering it, and adapted to the species and age of the animal.

Ella notices nothing, feels nothing, just slips away peacefully in her sleep. Tessa gives Ella another loving pat on her belly.

'Are you okay?' I ask when it's time to wrap up. I want to wait for Tessa, not rush anything.

'Sure, thank you. Carry on.'

Tessa leaves and Ella is moved with a crane to the hospital's post-mortem room, away from the other animals. I will examine her there, after which she will be stored in a large freezer room to be later safely disposed of.

During the post-mortem examination, I look for abscesses in the lungs, one of the symptoms of TB. But to my surprise, I find nothing. Once again, I send the blood samples to my contact at the Animal Health Agency for further testing, but they also come back positive. In the accompanying report of the BAL, however, I read that another bacterium was found: a mycobacterium that can give false positive results in TB tests. That's known in other animal species, but here that mycobacterium turns the whole story upside down. It's actually the first time this has been observed in pygmy hippos. This represents a breakthrough in the research on TB in pygmy hippos: because of that bacterium, the tests we normally use to detect the bacterium will not always give an accurate result. I immediately realize that this is huge; it should even be published. Normally, things that do not go as planned are not published, as is actually the case here. But that's exactly why this is such an interesting and educational case: all tests indicated that it was TB, even though that was probably not the case.

'Everyone always assumes that veterinarians can be wrong, but no one assumes that labs can also be wrong,' I say at the end of a follow-up meeting about Ella. I want to remind everyone in the team that nothing should be taken for granted and that mistakes can always occur.

After the meeting, Tessa takes me aside.

'Thank you,' she says. 'I still think we made the right decision with all the information we had.' I nod. That gratitude means a lot to me. Euthanasia of an animal should not become a habit or insensitive, though it is something I am gradually getting used to as a veterinarian. Simply because it is an almost daily part of my job. That may diminish the emotional weight, but the involvement remains significant. That's necessary, I believe. After all, the people around me are counting on me to do it properly. Regardless of the animal concerned, whether it's Ella with TB or a dog that has bitten its owner. Often I receive more gratitude for guiding people well and performing euthanasia properly than when I try to cure the animal in question. That's simply because the right decision is made by all the parties involved.

Outsiders might wonder if Ella ultimately died in vain. And it's a question I can understand. Ella is indeed an interesting case, as she was ultimately euthanized under the assumption that she had TB. Which we had not been able to confirm. So, probably unnecessary. Still, I hope I can provide an appropriate answer to that question by saying that Ella has contributed to science with her death. Thanks to her, our knowledge has expanded, which definitely gives her death meaning.

Marius

In 2014 there was a commotion. The headlines didn't beat around the bush: 'Zoo kills healthy giraffe' and 'Execution for giraffe Marius'.

The reality was, of course, more nuanced than those headlines would suggest.

Marius was born a year and a half earlier at Copenhagen Zoo, where the risk of inbreeding made him unsuitable for reproduction purposes. A move to another zoo was also not possible, according to the stud book, due to those genetic reasons, as a blood relationship between giraffes must always be avoided.

The zoo had no other choice but to not let the animal mature. Animal lovers had protested and raised many arguments to keep the animal alive. Many suggested castration, but that was not considered by the zoo because castration in this case could have too many adverse effects on his position in the group. Others suggested reintegration into the wild, but that generally has little chance of success and is not desired by the African countries where giraffes roam free.

The zoo has therefore made the best possible decision, in their case, taking all factors into account. An autopsy will be performed on Marius and then the carcass will be cut up to feed the predators. For that reason, he was killed with a pistol instead of an injection, as it would have contaminated the meat.

The decision to euthanize Marius was not much of an issue in Denmark itself, but in Belgium it had sparked a discussion about euthanasia, and in America they thought it was disgraceful. Whatever opinion one

holds, I think it is important to know the whole story before forming an opinion. Everything must be taken into account, starting with the EAZA network: the European network of zoos and aquariums.
Most good zoos are paying members of that organization and therefore have rights and obligations. One of those first important obligations is to apply for membership. This is done by filling out the application, with information about the correct number of animals present, the number of keepers, the number of visitors, the methods used for population management of the animals, the feeding policy, you name it. If that application is approved, the zoo undergoes a screening after which it is decided whether or not to accept it as EAZA member.
Zoos that are members can exchange animals for free among each other. To ensure that everything runs smoothly, a coordinator is appointed for each animal species, someone with specialized knowledge of the species who determines in which zoo animals live and whether or not they can be exchanged. The exchange programs fall under the European Endangered Species Program (EEP). The EEP establishes breeding programs to provide zoos with enough animals, so that these zoos do not have to take animals from the wild for their operation and population management. It mainly concerns endangered animal species, such as the gorilla or the Sumatran tiger. In this way, the genetic diversity of animal species is preserved. In practice, this means: a breeding group of elephants in a specific zoo receives breeding recommendations from the EEP coordinator for elephants. When an elephant has bred, it's decided to which zoo the calf

will be moved to or whether it can stay in the current group, depending on the sex, group dynamic, and genetic variability. The recommendations are adjusted every year, and to keep track each endangered animal has a stud book number. Animals that aren't endangered, like the plains zebra, the lion, or the springbok, don't have a stud book number but are managed by the zoo itself, because there's enough of them spread across all European zoos.

The ultimate goal of all these breeding programs is to avoid overbreeding, so that a certain species is not overrepresented. If that does happen, the zoo must make a decision according to the EAZA guidelines. According to those guidelines, the zoo is free to choose euthanasia, birth control, or export to another zoo when it comes to surplus animals.

If a particular zoo applies the 'breed and cull' strategy, it actually decides that the mother animals are allowed to breed, and the young will be raised by the mother just like in the wild until it is independent. In nature, the animal would eventually leave the nest or mother at a certain age to prevent inbreeding. In captivity, that is the moment to proceed with euthanasia. People sometimes wonder why those animals have to be born if they don't get to live long lives. The most important reason to choose this strategy is that breeding is the primary form of 'enrichment' for a mother animal and often an entire herd, as young animals are an important, dynamic part of the herd's structure. An additional reason is that these animals can then be fed to predators, as this strategy is primarily applied to herbivores. So it's a bit like the 'circle of life'. Because it's part of population management, EAZA doesn't condemn it. That often goes against public opinion, although deer that are euthanized and serve as food for lions and tigers are often not as notable to them as giraffes or elephants.

When a zoo chooses not to perform euthanasia, often because it doesn't align with the philosophy of a particular zoo or a particular culture, religion, or public opinion in a country, population management must be done through contraception or birth control. This way, isolation can prevent the animals from breeding. For solitary animals like felines, this is perfect, as this isolation has no impact on animal welfare. For other animals, it is possible to carry out temporary separation and remove the male from the group during the breeding season. A second option is a temporary sterilization of the male or female, which can be done by injecting various hormone preparations. There is even a European contraception group for zoos, where all information is collected. There is a risk that these hormone preparations can cause problems in the reproductive system, such as cancer and/or infections. This technique must therefore be closely monitored by a veterinarian. The final step is permanent sterilization. In that case, the female's ovaries are removed with or without the uterus, and the male undergoes castration, or a vasectomy if the group structure should not change. These animals are permanently eliminated from breeding, so this decision must be made very thoughtfully.

Each zoo is free to decide for themselves what to do with surplus animals for each animal group to maintain its population. That's what it ultimately comes down to. When the case of Marius was ongoing, my opinion was often asked for in the debate. That happens every time news of euthanasia in a zoo reaches the general public. So I'll give it here: I have worked both in zoos where they opt for the 'breed and cull' strategy and in zoos where they opt for breeding restrictions. With all that knowledge in mind, I understand both methods, as they each have their pros and cons.

The most beautiful and, at the same time, most painful incident involves the euthanasia of our own dog, who shared joys and sorrows with our family for fifteen years. The dog was sick and suffering unnecessarily, so as a family we made the decision together to put him out of his misery. I felt that I had to perform the euthanasia myself, with the help of my wife.

I gritted my teeth until he died, only to burst into tears together afterwards.

I wanted to support him, take responsibility and take care of him. And my wife and children assumed that I would do exactly that. I didn't want to disappoint them, just like I don't want to disappoint any animal.

11. Loss is also gain

Year of birth: 1993.
December 2005: blister on both front feet.
Treatment: trim hooves and administer anti-inflammatory medication. Successful.
I carefully review Garry's file, the onager I have to treat. Garry is the breeding male of our onager group. We're a year later and the wild donkey has been limping again for a while. The problem seems to be in both front legs, just like last year. To figure out what's going on, I need to sedate Garry. They're called wild donkeys for a reason, so Garry can't be examined without sedation.
I administer a sedative with the gun and when he is asleep, I can check his paws. Examining an onager or horse hoof is not that simple, since, like a blacksmith, I have to look inside the hoof to see if there's a problem. The main difference is that we cannot perform pain tests or check for a blister, as our onager is asleep and therefore does not feel any pain. That means I have to blindly search for a possible blister with a hoof knife. Finally, I find a large blister in both hooves. I take care of them by opening them. With a hissing sound, I hear the pressure escaping as the pus comes out. I'm clearly in the right place. I then need to sufficiently thin the hoof, so as to allow the blisters to heal. I also inject painkillers directly into the blood through the jugular vein, administer antibiotics in the gluteal muscles, and take a blood sample. The sample will be used for routine tests, but it remains to be seen whether that will provide information on why Garry is experiencing blisters for the second time.
However, the lab results come back normal, and yet Garry continues to limp. Because he is less mobile, the females are not so interested in him, and he is often alone.
So there is indeed more going on, which obliges me to consider the other options. First of all, I want to rule out laminitis, which is a metabolic disorder that disrupts the blood supply to the hoof. I start

the treatment, and two weeks later I check the hooves again. Once again I find myself on my knees in front of Garry. I immediately see that nothing has changed. On the contrary, there's even been some deterioration.

To confirm if it's laminitis, I proceed with an X-ray examination of the legs. This shows that there is indeed a rotation present in the coffin bone. Furthermore, hematology shows signs of inflammation. I also decide to measure the glucose level through a new blood sample, which could very well be the key to the solution. The values are indeed high, too high. That brings me to Cushing's disease. A long shot, since Cushing's is known in horses, but as yet not in wild donkeys.

The disease is caused by a dysfunction in a specific part of the brain. In Cushing's, a tumor is formed, causing a disturbance in the pituitary gland of the animal's brain. The pituitary gland starts to produce too much hormones, causing the adrenal gland to become overactive. So the problem is located in the brain, but it's actually an adrenal problem. The animal becomes hormonally imbalanced as a result, and in horses this manifests itself with a bloated belly, a curly coat, and therefore laminitis. When I take a closer look at my patient and compare him to his peers, I actually notice that his hair is curly and that he has a 'potbelly'. Could it really be this?

There's one more test necessary to confirm my suspicions that our Garry is indeed suffering from Cushing's: the dexamethasone suppression test. After administration of this corticosteroid preparation, there should be a clear decrease in the cortisol level in the blood of a healthy animal.

In Garry's case, this decrease is not present, confirming my suspicions. Garry has Cushing's disease.

I feel sorry for Garry, but at the same time I am proud of the research and the breakthrough. So Cushing's disease does indeed occur in wild donkeys as well. That means we can now treat Garry in a targeted manner. The treatment involves giving daily medication, which helps normalize the hormonal imbalance. Furthermore, we need to treat the symptoms, which means taking care of the blisters on the feet, and applying special casts to take pressure off the hoof and reverse the rotation of the coffin bone. It has to be done under anesthesia each time, four times every ten days. Garry also receives antibiotics, painkillers, and other medication for laminitis.

Slowly but surely, I see the blisters healing, but on closer inspection I notice that a deep wound has formed in the right foreleg all the way to the extensor tendon. Garry continues to deteriorate clinically. He also refuses to eat, not only causing his body weight to continue to decrease, but also preventing him from taking oral medication. The once beautifully muscular wild donkey has now become a skinny weak animal. It's heartbreaking to see.

We continue to treat the animal as best as possible, but a decision must be made three months after the diagnosis. The treatment is not effective because Garry does not want to take his medicine each day; the donkey's well-being is under a lot of pressure. It frustrates me enormously that I can't help the animal. It leaves me with a dilemma, now and in similar situations: should I continue to try to save the animal, or should I put it out of its misery? After discussion, everyone agrees: the only thing that can help is euthanasia.

I do consider the loss of Garry as a loss. Post-mortem examination should confirm that we made the right decision, and it indeed shows that the pituitary gland is enlarged bilaterally and that the adrenal glands are also enlarged. We have found the ultimate proof of Cushing's.

The death of this animal also brings some good, as we will be able to save other animals thanks to all the new information. After further investigation in archived samples of previous deaths of onagers, we can even confirm another animal with Cushing's through histopathological examination. It is thanks to this research that our Garry is now referenced in the literature and that Cushing's disease is now known to occur among wild equids.

12. Damned if you do and damned if you don't

I stare out of a small window on the boat. The only thing I see is water, in front of me, behind me, to my left and to my right. The sky is gray and it's foggy, so visibility is limited.

'Boat!' 'Boat!' cooed Jef, who is just learning his first words.

'The boat is sailing,' Jonah adds.

We are on our way back to our house in England, after a weekend in Belgium. It feels good to see family and friends again, but I always look forward to returning to our life in England.

'Tim! A call...' Marie hands me my ringing cell phone.

'Amilia is sick,' I'm told straightaway. It's Lee, the keeper of Amilia, our TWO-AND-HALF-year-old elephant.

I curse under my breath.

'What are the symptoms?'

'During the walk through the park, she didn't hold her mother's tail, which she normally always does.'

It may seem like a small detail, but I trust Lee when he thinks something is not right.

I immediately look at my watch. We still have to sail on the boat for an hour and then drive for another two hours to reach the zoo.

'I'll be there as soon as I can.'

Three hours later I arrive at Amilia's side. Lee immediately provides an update.

'At first glance, everything seems fine, but I don't trust it.'

'I need to check her tongue,' I say to Lee, who immediately helps me position Amilia in front of me. She stands up straight and Lee asks her to open her mouth, which she has been trained to do.

'And?' he asks when I stay silent for too long while looking at that tongue.

'Do you see this, those blue spots? That means she has pinpoint bleeding.'

I curse again. Loudly, this time.
'I fear it's herpes,' I say when I notice Lee looking at me expectantly and fearfully.
Endotheliotropic Elephant Herpes, or EEHV for short, is a virus that can kill an elephant in 24 to 48 hours.
There are different herpes viruses circulating among elephants, but EEHV does not cause cold sores in the oral cavity like herpes in humans. It is one of the main causes of mortality in young Asian elephants, both in the wild and in zoos. We currently don't know much about the virus, except that it is latent in most elephants. Young animals are particularly susceptible to it. The virus causes an acute bleeding disease, leading to internal bleeding in the animal. A part of the blood vessels becomes as leaky as a sieve, causing all the blood to leave the bloodstream and the animal to bleed to death internally. It's similar to what rat poison does to a rat. Young Asian elephants die in more than 80 percent of cases after just a few hours or days once the first clinical symptoms become noticeable.
Lee is silent, waiting for more explanation.
'The fact that she is not holding her tail with her trunk means she has been sick longer than we could have suspected.'
'If only I had…'
'No. The first few days usually slip past us. You couldn't have noticed anything different or earlier than what you've already seen.' I want to reassure him, because he is not to blame. This virus first multiplies locally, probably in the upper respiratory tract, before rampaging in the blood a few days later. The primary phase is not noticeable in elephants, so by the time we notice symptoms, we are already in the secondary phase. By then, the virus may have already caused a lot of damage, significantly reducing the chances of saving the animal.
'Okay,' Lee says doggedly. 'What can we do? What treatment can we start?'
'I don't know...' I say in all honesty. If Amilia does indeed have the herpes virus, she would be the first elephant in England. And I the first in England to fight that virus. Something that has never been successful to my knowledge.

'You're damned if you do and you're damned if you don't,' I say. 'That's what it comes down to.' If we do nothing, Amilia will die anyway. But if we do something, there's no guarantee she will survive.

'Are you sure?' Lee asks again.

I nod. I can take a blood test, but there are no reference laboratories in England, so we cannot get an immediate analysis.

'I'll start by administering an anti-inflammatory agent and anti-herpes medication, but I can't guarantee it will help.' The virus is undetectable in elephants, so we also don't know if the medicine will help, but it's the best option.

'We'll also start fluid therapy.'

'Sounds good,' Lee nods. Amilia and her mother are isolated from the group so we can treat her in peace. We place an IV in a blood vessel of the ear and start administering the fluid.

Meanwhile, we ask Amilia again to open her mouth, and we now see that the pinpoint bleedings are getting larger and that there is also more bleeding.

That night, together with Lee, I keep watch over Amilia.

'It's unbelievable how ferocious that nasty virus is,' he says softly.

I nod. The realization that we have no certainty of a cure is now also sinking in with Lee. It's a gamble. Fingers crossed.

'Why does it have to be so damn fast, too? This morning there was nothing wrong. And now...' Lee visibly struggles and I also have a lump in my throat. It's terrible to see an animal die, because that is what's happening here. An elephant is such a mighty, powerful, intelligent animal. It shouldn't die from some stupid elusive virus.

The next morning, Adam, Don, and Andy arrive for their day's work.

'Are you okay?'

'No,' says Lee.

'No,' I agree.

Amilia's tongue is now clearly swollen and completely blue. Her head and lower abdomen are also swollen due to the edemas that are forming.

We all continue to silently watch Amilia for a while. Five men, usually not shy of showing off their bravado, but now cracked by powerlessness and sadness.

We work through the day sharing very few words, and continue into the night. Amilia's condition has deteriorated further and she can no longer stand on her legs. She is having difficulty breathing. The IV is still running and we continue the treatment, not wanting to give up, against our better judgment. A few hours later, I have to break the silence by saying something everyone already knows.
'She has passed away.' Amilia lost the battle 48 hours after the onset of the first symptoms. It's the first time I see a group of men cry.

And it's the first time I join in crying, out of sadness, out of anger, but mostly out of powerlessness, powerlessness against this damn virus that can kill such a beautiful, majestic elephant in just a few days.

Unfortunately, the work doesn't stop here. I have to conduct a post-mortem examination now, no matter how difficult it may be at this moment. As a veterinarian, I realize of course that this research is invaluable, because it will teach me what exactly the virus does to the organs of the animal. This way, hopefully, in the future, I will be able to treat other elephants better.
What I see is hard to describe: there are two liters of fluid between the heart and the pericardium, the sac containing the heart. The heart has extensive bleeding throughout the heart wall. There is extensive pulmonary edema. The gastrointestinal system has pinpoint bleeding throughout its entire length. The spleen has doubled in size and is extremely swollen. It is clear to me that all the fluid we have given has flowed out of the bloodstream into the peripheral tissues, and that our elephant was doomed at that point. 'It was like pouring water into a broken bucket,' I grumble disappointedly.
With Amilia, we did not have much knowledge about any possible treatment. Unfortunately, after Amilia, we also lost Bets and Riddle, which makes three young elephants in five years. The only positive

thing about this is that we have learned something new each time, especially about the correct fluid therapy and the prognosis or outcome based on the blood tests. Meanwhile, years later, much more knowledge has been gained. I can now look back on all the cases myself, including two elephants that I did manage to save. I can say that as a veterinarian I can help an elephant get through it, but at the same time I am convinced that the elephant itself plays a role in overcoming the disease. There is something that makes one survive while the other does not. The number of white blood cells can be an indication: a high number of white blood cells indicates the development of a response against the virus. A low number of white blood cells indicates the absence of that immune response. By looking at the blood, a prediction can be made about whether the elephant will survive or not. There's currently a vaccine in the works, but there is no guarantee of its effectiveness yet. Anyway, we are all convinced: we are going to teach that f*cking virus a lesson. Even if just to honor Amilia, Bets, and Riddle.

13. That's what I'm aiming for

On the examination table lies Suki, a red panda. Suki lives here in Whipsnade in a beautiful enclosure. There's an island surrounded by water and large trees, and he has the company of a female and two cubs. Usually he is very active and playful, but now he is lying drowsy and sleepy on the table.

'I found him this morning on the floor of his enclosure,' explains Marc, one of his keepers. 'It seems like he has lost all interest and energy.'

It's indeed not normal for him to be this weak. Suki is a red panda, a mustelid that eats only bamboo, and enjoys playing in the trees. It's a curious little creature.

I run my hand over Suki's fur and notice that he has bald patches here and there. I immediately feel how skinny he is.

'I can count his ribs,' I say worriedly to Marc. 'His hip bones are sticking out.'

Marc nods concerned.

I take Suki's temperature and the thermometer reads 'low temperature'.

'Darn it...' I mumble. 'Hypothermia symptoms. He is also dehydrated. Look...'

I pinch Suki's skin, which stays upright instead of folding back. Suki lets it all happen and looks back at us pitifully.

'He needs warm liquid,' I say quickly. 'Let's start with that.'

I search in vain for a vein that is easy for a needle.

'Subcutaneous it is then,' I decide. This way, his body can absorb the liquid, which will help him rehydrate and warm up.

He doesn't respond to what I am doing, that's how weak he is.

'We can't do anything else now,' I conclude. 'I'll let him warm up further by putting him in a small enclosure with a heat lamp. I'll also fill rubber gloves with warm water to place against him, like a hot water bottle.'

Marc slips away, I feel sorry for him.
'I'll call you as soon as there's any change.'
I monitor Suki for an hour, and slowly but surely I see improvement. Where just a moment ago he lay motionless on the table, he now starts to move a little. So it seems to be helping. It takes a while each time, but after first moving his head and lifting it up, he now also starts crawling around. Eventually, he even regains enough strength in his legs to push himself up and waddle around in his hospital enclosure.
'There is life in him again,' I tell Marc on the phone. We are about two hours later and Suki seems to have recovered a bit.
'I'll be right there,' he replies.
'I've noticed some weakness in his hindquarters,' I say. 'And he's making uncoordinated movements with his hind legs. Something is definitely not right. The bald patches in his fur also worry me,' I note. Marc nods and seems relieved that I don't simply dismiss his findings. On the contrary, I take everything a keeper points out seriously, as they know their animal best. They can even notice the smallest change in behavior or appearance. Changes that wouldn't stand out to me as a veterinarian, simply because I don't know the animal well enough.
'Can you do more now?' Marc asks, to which I look at Suki for a second. He may be a bit more lively again, but I don't want to burden him any more now.
'Tomorrow,' I say. 'Then I will put him in his crate under sedation for further examination.'
The next day I can just pick him up again. He's not running, not playing, he just let's me do what I want. Still, it strikes me again how skinny he is, and the scale confirms it. Suki currently weighs 11 pounds, while this should easily be around 22 pounds. There's clearly reduced muscle mass in the hindquarters, and the bilateral alopecia, or hair loss, on both hind flanks is hard to ignore.
I review my differential diagnoses once again, the list of all conditions that could be relevant here. I rule out some options, such as parasites and fungal infection. In the end, I am left with Addison's

disease, which is caused by an inflammation of the adrenal glands. But this would be new territory for red pandas. Because of the hair loss, I also consider a hormonal problem: hypothyroidism, where a slow-working thyroid causes an animal to become sluggish, walk stiffly, and lie down to sleep in a warm place. Just like Suki is doing. But hypothyroidism, which is mainly seen in dogs, usually leads to weight gain, and that's not the case with Suki. Moreover, the condition has never been described in the literature when it comes to red pandas, except in one animal where this was suggested post-mortem. After the differential diagnosis, I decide to put Suki under gas anesthesia and continue my examination. His heart, lungs, organs... everything seems fine.

I then focus further on the hair loss. With my fingers, I run through the fur again and check for bald spots. The skin is not red and does not feel warm, so I can rule out any primary inflammation of bacterial origin. A skin cell test also yields nothing. I also don't suspect a parasitic cause, as Suki would then be itching from fleas or mites. A fungal infection also looks different. That brings me back to my initial thought, a hormonal cause. I collect a blood sample and request hormonal tests in addition to the routine examination. The thyroid and adrenal glands need to be examined.

When the blood test results come back, I find the missing piece of the puzzle: Suki has a low level of T4 or thyroxine, the thyroid hormone. A problem with the thyroid would therefore be a logical explanation, especially with the hair loss, although other diseases can also cause a decrease in thyroid hormone. To confirm my suspicions, I still need to do an additional test, the TSH stimulation test, which does confirm the hypothyroidism diagnosis.

I immediately pick up the phone and call Marc again.

'Marc... I got it. A hormonal issue that has never been discovered before in a living red panda.'

'Oh no...' Marc sighs.

But...,' I say loudly and clearly, 'that doesn't mean it can't be treated successfully. Because that's what I'm aiming for.'

I start a treatment with synthetic thyroid hormone and levothyroxine, and Suki is monitored daily. After two weeks, an improvement in his behavior is visible. With a smile, I watch as Suki responds in his enclosure the way he should. The weakness in his hindquarters has gone and he runs over the branches as if nothing is wrong. He becomes more active and responds increasingly to the keepers and his environment. Hair growth also increases again.

I evaluate the treatment over time and after two months Suki is back on his feet. His fur is shiny again like before, and all the bald spots are gone. However, he does now suffer from a chronic illness, but it is perfectly manageable in this way.

My goal has been achieved. A new disease has been identified in this animal species and it is possible to treat that disease. For the first time.

I end up talking about Suki at a conference in England, because it's a case report that's important enough to share with my colleagues, if they were ever to encounter this in one of their animals as well. And hopefully this lecture could, somewhere, save a panda suffering from this disease. While I'm giving my presentation, I look at the photos of Suki passing by on the big screen. The contrast between that weak, sick red panda and the vibrant version afterwards is huge. But I notice something else. In photos which show Marc, you can almost see how heavy the burden on his shoulders is. His body language, his gaze, his demeanor... The contrast between that worried keeper and the reassured version afterwards is enormous. I really didn't realize it at the time, but that's what I'm aiming for as well.

14. As it should be

The old Landrover Jeep rattles as we drive through the zoo. My nurse is driving and I'm holding onto the door handle with one hand. The vibe in the jeep is fantastic. We're on our way to Kuna, one of our Indian rhinos who is about to give birth. Her calf will be the first Indian rhino calf to be born here at Whipsnade Zoo, so it's a special event in so many ways. At the box, not accessible to the public, we are greeted by Roger and Shiobhan, Kuna's regular keepers, who have been observing her from a distance via a camera for a while.

Once we join them, I do my check, as far as possible on that small TV screen: Kuna looks good, her breathing seems under control, and she shows no signs of weakness or drowsiness. Her pregnant belly is huge, so after a pregnancy of sixteen months, she will soon finally be relieved and carry a whopping 220 pounds less weight all at once. Not that a rhino calf weighs 220 pounds; they weigh around 90 pounds, but the amniotic fluid around the baby and the placenta can easily weigh 110 to 130 pounds together.

Kuna walks around a bit nervously, but still has maintained her powerful aura. She has a certain determination, despite or perhaps thanks to the effort that awaits her. I observe her breathing, which is deep and regular. Her movements resemble a kind of swaying. She pushes the straw on the ground of her stall aside with her snout, so she can lie down more easily, and then lowers herself onto her side. It won't be long now.

Nobody dares breaking the silence, I think they're even holding their breath.

Kuna pauses for a moment before she starts pushing. It's difficult for her, but slowly but surely we see the amniotic sac appear. Kuna stands up and her water breaks with a big splash. She spins around a few times and then lies down again and pushes once more. We see two little feet appear, hind feet. Kuna gets up again, and gravity does the rest as the calf falls to the ground with a thud. Talk about a grand entrance!

'Wow...' Shiobhan is impressed. Everyone is impressed, and we all start hugging and congratulating each other. We have just became uncles and aunts!

'Perfect,' I say under my breath. We don't have to intervene and that's perfect, the way it should be. There are certain protocols we must follow during the birth of large animals, but the most important thing is always: do not intervene unless necessary. And that seems to be the case here fortunately.

While the calf remains lying on the ground and makes a few cautious movements, Kuna turns to her calf and nudges it with her snout, then carefully licks her clean.

Shiobhan lets out an 'Ohhh...' It's a beautiful spectacle, there's nothing as powerful as that maternal instinct. After about ten minutes, the calf gets up, supported by Kuna. The first steps of the newborn animal are hesitant and endearing, and are all captured on our phone cameras.

'Welcome, Aisha!' whoops Shiobhan, immediately joined by colleague Roger.

'Or Raja!' he corrects. We, in fact, don't yet know if it's a male or a female.

But Shiobhan doesn't even hear him. 'They left,' she concludes.

I agree. 'As it should be.'

Except for watching the calf quietly discover the world all day, I can't do much else at the moment. We need to stay away from the mother and child for as long as possible, so they can rely on their instincts and find their own way. The most important thing to monitor now is whether the calf is nursing from the mother. That's essential.

'I'll let you know if there are any complications,' I say. 'Watch the drinking, hey.' After that, Jo and I leave for the hospital, totally at ease now, as we talk to each other about what we had just experienced, reliving every moment. Indeed, emotions can sometimes run high when witnessing something so rare and beautiful. I don't expect any further issues now and feel the adrenaline draining from my body.

However, a few hours later I get a call from Shiobhan.
'The calf hasn't drunk yet,' she says. She sounds worried. It's not a disaster that it hasn't drunk yet, but it's definitely something to keep an eye on. The calf should be able to drink from the mother on its own within a few hours of birth. The colostrum is pretty much vital for the newborn. It is the mother's first milk that is released and helps strengthen the calf's immune system. Calves are born without protective immunity against infectious disease organisms. Therefore, they need a passive transfer of infection-fighting proteins, called antibodies, found in the mother's first milk, colostrum. Antibodies are transferred to the calf from the mother in the first 12 hours after birth. If the calf does not receive colostrum, it's not protected against viruses and bacteria. This is called failure of passive transfer (FPT), where animals are at risk of developing serious medical conditions. We need to try to avoid that.
I decide to take another look myself and I notice that the calf is indeed instinctively searching for Kuna's teats, but is unable to drink. It pushes its snout under Kuna's bulky body, but it doesn't get any further than some bumping and pushing.
We don't know why yet, but when a calf does not drink from the mother on its own, there are usually two main causes. Which immediately leads me to a differential diagnosis: either the calf isn't smart or strong enough to find the milk, or Kuna has a problem and won't allow the calf to drink because of it. For example, this could be painful swelling of the udder, a wound on the nipple causing pain, or simply the inexperience of the mother, turning around every time the calf tries to drink.
'Shall we see what the protocol suggests?' asks my nurse Jo. 'We could perhaps feed it additional milk?'
'Is supplemental feeding actually a good idea, though?' I wonder out loud It's the first question I have to answer. It is known that animals raised by hand-rearing often exhibit more aggressive behavior towards humans later on. Especially with males. Through intensive contact with people during those feedings, they become familiar with them and lose their natural fear. That's in contrast to animals that

are not hand-reared. The distance to humans is naturally greater for them, causing them to have a certain fear and keep their distance. If we do proceed with hand-rearing where we supplement the calf's food, we also need a certain type of milk. We can't just pick those up at the supermarket: they need to be carefully put together and that takes time.

'It's been six hours already,' Shiobhan says. She keeps her eyes on the calf that continues to struggle, providing the strongest argument to start supplementary feeding.

'Two more hours without food and the calf will start to weaken,' I agree.

What should I do?

I organize my thoughts and go back to the most important rule when a calf is born: we only take the calf away from the mother if all other options fail.

So I go over those options. With a horse, I would lead the foal to the mother, hold it and let it drink. I would also touch the mare's udder to make sure she is not in pain. But that is impossible with a rhino. Still, I must find a way to try and see where the problem lies, the calf or the mother.

'I'm going to sedate Kuna,' I decide. She has just given birth and will want to protect her calf at all costs, so she will not tolerate any visitors in their enclosure. Therefore, she must first be sedated so that her calf can be examined and then returned to her. By combining two sedatives, I can ensure that Kuna does not fall to the ground, but still stays upright. That should work. Sedating large animals is my specialty and I have developed a protocol for it that is used worldwide. But it remains to be seen whether the calf is able to do what I want it to do.

I shoot a dart behind Kuna's ear, because the skin everywhere else is too thick to penetrate. We then wait twenty minutes, the time needed for the sedative to take effect. When I'm sure Kuna won't react aggressively to our presence, I enter the box first. It's actually a dark stable that isn't very big, which also doesn't give me much confidence as I step inside. Kuna and her calf may be considered cute, but they are still huge animals that can be very aggressive when they feel

threatened. I take a first step into the box and immediately feel the adrenaline rushing through my body. I feel my heart pounding in my throat. My heart is racing as I try to focus on my breathing. I cautiously step towards Kuna, she looks at me dully with her big, dark eyes and I ignore the hesitation I feel. I carefully reach out my hand and manage to blindfold her. With the blindfold, Kuna can no longer see where we are moving around her, making it safer for those in the box. I signal that Jo and Shiobhan can also come in. They will first look at the calf. It must be checked for hypothermia and they also have to see that it has enough strength to continue searching for the nipples. The temperature is measured rectally and it's okay. The calf is already trying to give Jo and Shiobhan headbutts with its non-existent horn, so it is definitely still strong enough.
'It's a boy!' Jo says, quickly doing a check. 'Hi, little Raja.'
Meanwhile, I examine Kuna. I immediately check her udder. That doesn't feel hard, isn't swollen, and doesn't seem painful. When I milk her, milk even comes out. I don't want that colostrum to go to waste, so Jo collects the milk and feeds it to the calf right away with a bottle, which eagerly swallows it. A relief. The longer the young calf does not drink, the more dangerous. Also, the fact that Kuna can provide that milk is nothing but positive. The first two days she will only produce around 10 ounces of milk, to produce larger quantities on day three. To make that process successful, it's important to stimulate milk production by allowing the calf to drink or by milking her. So that's what I'm going to do. It sounds simpler than it is. A rhino has very short nipples, making milking tricky. The milk sprays in all directions and drips down her belly over her thick legs.
'The milk is definitely not the problem,' I remark amused. It's reassuring, that's for sure. While I milk Kuna, Emma catches everything to pour it into a feeding bottle.
Finally, we manage to collect and give 3.5 ounces of colostrum to Raja, without any additional feeding. I only administer some ORS through the bottle as well. It's an oral rehydration solution that should ensure he continues to have enough energy.
'Let's give it a try,' I say to Shiobhan and Jo. I want to bring Raja

to Kuna to help him drink. The three of us try to move Raja, but he resists. He's headbutting, almost pushing us over, and is simply way too wild. It's becoming too much trouble.
Raja barely reaches just below my knee, but has the attitude of a 7,000-pound rhino.
'Be careful with Kuna!' Jo remarks.

My gaze shifts from Raja to Kuna, and despite the sedation and the fact that she can't see anything because of her blindfold, she becomes restless. She positions herself to defend herself and her young, which also seems ready for a confrontation.

'We'll stop now,' I decide. 'The colostrum has been drunk, the ORS has been administered, and they are both healthy. They will get through the night. If necessary, we can sedate and milk Kuna again tomorrow. As long as we can avoid hand-rearing.'
I inject Kunba with something to counteract the sedation, remove the blindfold from her eyes and then we all make a run for it. We watch from a safe distance again. Raja seems to need to recover from the adventure, and Kuna also looks a bit confused; but after a few minutes, she walks determinedly towards her calf. Raja starts searching for milk on his own again. His little head pushes and shoves under that big belly again, but, once more, it doesn't seem to work. Until he turns his head a little and licks Kuna's paws with his tongue.
'Look now,' I say surprised.
Raja is licking more eagerly at those paws, which the drops of milk flowed on when I milked her.
'He's following the trail...' Jo says with admiration.
The drops naturally guide Raja towards the nipples, where he eventually starts drinking. Raja has found the way. Not with crumbs like in that fairy tale, but with drops.

15. Understanding for the lack of understanding

Jonah, our oldest son of three years, is playing quietly, while one-year-old Jef has just woken up from a nap. It's Sunday, so we mostly try to do nothing. Family obligations are not something we have here in Whipsnade, although we do regularly meet up with our new friends. Since we're a family of five, it's also nice to just be at home and enjoy each other's company. Marie often takes care of the children here on her own while I work at the zoo, so it's nice for everyone to be together on the weekends.

Although the weekend is no guarantee of free time.

'The zoo!' Marie shouts while answering the ringing phone. She's holding Jef with one arm, while she hands me the phone with the other.

She looks at curiously me while I'm on the phone. A call like this on the weekend is rarely good news, as we already know, and Marie suspects that now as well. And she's right.

'A Milu deer that can't give birth,' I apologize as I hang up. But Marie shakes her head, laughing.

'No worries, we'll come with you.' Marie and the children often come with me to the zoo when I get called in on weekends. That way, we can make the best of a bad situation and carry on spending the afternoon with the children.

On the way to the zoo, I try to explain the problem, but a giggling Jef and a chatty Jonah in the backseat prevent any adult conversation. So I keep it short.

'Milu deer tend to have difficult deliveries, usually because of the calf's poor positioning. That's probably the case now as well.'

'Uh huh,' mumbles Marie, who's turned around in the passenger seat searching for Jef's pacifier.

Once arrived, we get in the Land Rover and hurry to the enclosure of the Pere David's deer. These deer live together with the camels and yaks in a large enclosure visitors can drive through by car. Beautiful for the visitors, but not the easiest place to deliver a calf. The animals associate the Land Rover with 'bad news' so keep their distance. I leave the Land Rover at the entrance and tell Marie that I will call her when she can drive to me. I get into the car with keeper Chrissy and we hit the road. The animals recognize this car as 'food', so I can get relatively close to the deer. I shoot a dart in the deer's hindquarters from the passenger seat and call Marie to come closer. Once the deer is asleep, we drive over and park the cars so the visitors can't see what I'm doing and I won't get distracted. I unload my 'emergency kit' from the car and put on my delivery coat. After that, I get to work while Marie watches with Jef in her arms, who is falling asleep again. Jonah is busy supervising the procedure. He's a complete animal freak.

I first disinfect the vulva of the deer, followed by my hands. I apply some lubricant to my left arm and slide it inside the vagina, through the cervix into the uterus.

'Okay, I can feel it now. It's a compound shoulder presentation,' I say. 'This calf would never come out like this.'

In a shoulder presentation, both front legs are positioned backwards. I grab the first leg at the bottom, push it upwards, and then pull it forward. There we go. The first leg is in place. I do the same for the second leg. Now both legs are next to the head in the birth canal. It's now just a matter of carefully pulling the calf out, and that goes very smoothly. When the calf is out, I take a syringe and proceed with euthanasia. I wake the mother by injecting an antibody and she walks back into the group a bit dazed.

Some time later I'm next to Marie again. I notice she's standing there hesitantly, looking a bit nervous.

'What did you just do?' she asks immediately.

'What do you mean?'

'Did you euthanize that fawn? Or not?'

'Yes,' I nod, unaware of any wrongdoing.

'But why? That wasn't even necessary?'

Her lack of understanding makes me realize I didn't get the chance to give the full explanation on my way here. I not only had to help the deer give birth, but I also had to euthanize the calf. I knew that in advance. But for Marie, it came as a surprise. An unpleasant surprise.

'But it was,' I explain. 'If a deer like this cannot give birth naturally without our help, the calf cannot survive. The mother simply wouldn't accept it and might even kill it herself. First of all, because our scent is on the calf, but also because she was under anesthesia during the procedure and therefore doesn't know this is her young. So this is the best option for the calf.'

Marie looks surprised, which in turn surprises me as well. She knows how things are done in a zoo. She understands the principle of euthanasia, and also understands that this option is not chosen lightly. There's always a valid reason for killing an animal, otherwise we would never do it.

'But can't you just hand-rear the fawn?'

'No, because hand-rearing deer almost always goes wrong. Once they're independent, it's impossible to reintroduce them to the group. By then, the animals think they're human.'

'So then keep it separated? Raise it separately?'

'That wouldn't improve its quality of life, would it? Deer are social animals. It also often happens that these animals lose their fear of humans and often become aggressive when they are adults. This wouldn't be the first deer to push a keeper to the ground and injure them,' I say.

Marie tightens her grip around Jef, who has woken up from our argument. She's really upset. I haven't seen her like this very often. Not when it comes to my work.

'Marie,' I ask. 'Surely, you aren't against euthanasia? You've always understood why it's done, right?'

'Always, but not right now,' she answers sternly. 'I thought I came here to watch the birth of a little deer. But instead I get this shoved in my face. I'll understand soon enough, but give me time to process it all, okay.'

‘I know,’ I reply. And I trust that Marie will not blame me for doing my job as well as possible. 'I should have explained it better.'
I realize that Marie currently represents a large part of public opinion, to which we will always have to justify ourselves. Something we will continue to do, out of understanding for the lack of understanding.

2011-2013: Al Wabra Wildlife Preservation, Qatar

Although England was fantastic when it comes to veterinary care, I still wanted to develop further in the zoo world. Internally, there were no opportunities, so I started looking elsewhere for other options. In Qatar there was a private zoo run by a German veterinarian who apparently had moved back to Germany. On the website of the zoo, I found the job offer to become the director of Al Wabra Wildlife Preservation. I talked about it with Marie and was given her blessing to go and take a look at the zoo. The setup of this zoo was similar to that of Abu Dhabi, although everything was done at a smaller scale. The animal species were even more special and rare, especially the Spix's macaw, the birds of paradise, the gerenuk, and the beira antelope. The opportunity to run a zoo and manage people really appealed to me. So Marie and I decided together to move back to the Middle East.

I was, and still am today, a true mammal guy. That's why the antelopes and gazelles attracted me the most, but it quickly became clear that the Spix's macaw was the most important animal in this zoo. I quickly educated myself in the field of avian veterinary medicine and in the history of the Spix's macaw.

The sheikh and owner of Al Wabra was without a doubt the most visionary person I have ever met. I will probably never meet someone like that again. He

knew everything about the most endangered animal and plant species and wanted to save what he could. Before it was too late. So not only did he have extremely rare animals to breed, he also had the rarest and most endangered cicadas in his collection in order to protect them. When I sat with him in his majilis, a kind of meeting space, on a Friday, I hung on his every word so as not to miss any detail of his stories.
I was allowed to travel to countries I had never even heard of before, such as Djibouti, on his behalf to protect animals I had never heard of before, such as the dibatag.
Within two years I had traveled through a large part of Africa and Brazil to help protect animals. My air miles went through the roof.
Meanwhile, the three children attended the International School in Doha and made friends from different backgrounds. It was enormously enriching for them, and Marie was the glue that held everyone together.

16. Do or die: Spix's macaw part 1

The Spix's macaw collection at AWWP is exceptional, as it is an extremely endangered species. The parrot has even become extinct in the wild. That's because the Spix's macaw has fallen victim to poachers. The last specimen was literally plucked from the nest. Added to this is the illegal trade in the birds, while their habitat in the Brazilian Caatinga is being destroyed by changing agricultural techniques, where goats, sheep, and cows eat the food trees so crucial for the species. The Caatinga is a semi-desert, meaning that for most of the year it's very dry with no rain, and that, during the short rainy season, it rains a lot in a few months, turning it green. In the past, dams were built in the Caatinga, albeit not watertight, with branches, trees, mud and so on. They were supposed to slow down the water and keep it pooled as long as possible, maximizing the greenery. But because animals destroy and eat these dams, there is much less water. In 2000, the last Spix's macaw disappeared, making the species extinct in the wild. At that time, there were still about 60 Spix's macaws living in captivity, although mostly illegally. Sheikh Saoud Bin Mohammed Bin Ali Thani, owner of AWWP, then began a sort of last-chance rescue operation. He collected a number of Spix's macaws that were scattered among individuals worldwide and housed them in Qatar in a state-of-the-art breeding center. Caring for the birds is literally and figuratively a matter of life and death, as is managing their genetic heritage. If we want to prevent the birds from going extinct completely, we must preserve the genetic diversity as much as possible. There is so much going on around those animals that they actually take up my entire workday.

The moment I start in AWWP, the Spix's macaw is already being bred, although not much. When I check the data in the studbook, it quickly becomes clear that it is always the same couples that are

breeding, and that there's a lot of inbreeding. There are also a lot of infertile eggs. Each breeding season, only three to four offspring are born. When the females do lay eggs, they are most definitely fertile, so the problem must lie with the males. Due to poor breeding, inbreeding, and a high prevalence of diseases, the population is increasing far too slowly. It's clearly going through a genetic bottleneck. It's called that because you can really visualize that you have many animals in the bottle, but only a few come out on the other side due to the narrowing in the neck. If this lasts, your species will go extinct.
I sit with Cromwell, the South African parrot specialist who takes care of the Spix's macaws daily, to see what we can do.
'If this were a mammal, I would carry out artificial insemination,' I say.
'Why don't we do that then?' he asks. 'It happens quite often with parrots, no?.'
'Okay, I didn't know that. If that's the case, then let's do it, because it's really 'do or die' for our macaws. And as long as I'm here, it definitely won't be 'die'.
We end up finding a German veterinary team specialized in artificial insemination for parrots. Daniel, a young veterinarian, first started experimenting with his own parrots and then with those of customers. He designed a special device to insert into the cloaca of the parrot and induce ejaculation with electric shocks. I call him and he is immediately willing to come to Qatar and work with the Spix's macaw.
'We're waiting for the female to lay her first egg,' Daniel explains. 'Because we have to ensure the sperm fertilizes the egg before the eggshell is formed; this way, we are sure to be on time for the second and third eggs.'
'We'll collect sperm from all the males and check which sperm is of good quality, and then you can see, based on the studbook, which sperm we can use for each individual female.'
It's really fascinating to me, as a big mammal guy, to see a specialized veterinarian working on such a rare and small bird. Cromwell holds the parrot, and Daniel inserts the tiny probe into the cloaca. He carefully turns the knob of the electro-ejaculator to stimulate

it with electric shocks. After that, he massages the sperm into a pipette.

For the first time in my life, I see sperm cells of Spix's macaws moving under the microscope. I get an immediate sense that we might be working on something big here. It even gives me goosebumps, and that from a bird no less.

Now we wait for a female to lay an egg, and then we can repeat the whole process with the right male and inseminate her.

'B18,' says Cromwell. 'The female in B18 has laid an egg.'

We spring straight into action. First, we collect sperm from the genetically best male and then we go to her nest box. Cromwell catches her carefully and holds her tight. Daniel inserts the pipette with sperm into the cloaca and inseminates the first Spix's macaw ever. We put her back without exchanging any words and look at each other hopefully. This procedure is repeated a few more times before Daniel leaves us again.

The eggs of Spix's macaws are artificially incubated because due to their rarity, we cannot risk a female breaking her eggs. After an egg is laid, we replace it with a plastic replica and put the precious egg in the incubator.

A few days later, Cromwell and I are standing at the incubator rather nervously. We're going to candle the eggs today. We shine a light through the egg and see if an embryo is developing. That's always exciting, but today more than ever, because these are the eggs from artificial insemination. Carefully, we take the little egg and shine light on the shell: 'YES!!' we both say at the same time. We clearly see blood vessels in the egg, so we're sure that something is growing. We carefully place our 'world premiere' back in the incubator and hold each other tightly. We're both emotional. In the end, two chicks are born in the first year through the artificial insemination of couples who have never reproduced before. Every following year, there are a couple more as we escape out of that genetic bottleneck. Phase 1 of saving this species has succeeded.

17. This may sting for a moment

I step away from our research station. A base camp without running water or electricity, it is located a three hour drive from the nearest village, which can only be reached by a 4x4 vehicle. I'm in the tropical rain forest of Ivory Coast in West Africa, and not for leisure. I am here as a part of a project with pygmy hippos, where we want to study these animals in the wild to find out why they produce more female than male sperm. I'm accompanied by two doctoral students and some locals who are assisting us. There's also a three-man BBC film crew with us making a documentary.

Waving my arms, I brush the branches and leaves away from my face. I want to go out on my own for a bit, because if I don't, I might go completely nuts in this rain forest. The scorching heat, humidity, the buckets of rain... It's hard for me to get used to these conditions. Not to mention the thousands of mosquitoes. Carrying malaria of course. But it's that frustration that teaches me how overwhelming nature is. It's a jungle full of life with an enormous biodiversity, a place where you feel incredibly small as a human. Mother nature is in charge. Different rules apply here than in the zoo. In a zoo, a kind of artificial climate is created to the best possible extent, so that each animal can thrive in the best possible conditions. That seems to work well for me too. In that limited animal world, I know perfectly well how and what to do. In the wild, however, things are somewhat different, as I am experiencing again in this rain forest.

I close my eyes and try to take in the moment. This way, I hear the relentless sounds filling the jungle even more. I recognize the sound of crickets, birds, the wind, and the screeching of monkeys in the distance.

The research is not progressing very smoothly, as we have not been able to catch a pygmy hippopotamus yet. Today's only loot is hippo poop.

In the evening, I'm playing a card game with the two students when one of the locals runs towards us in a panic.
'Doctor! he calls out hurriedly. 'Doctor, you need to come with me! We have a problem!'
I'm startled and immediately all sorts of doomsday scenarios flash through my mind. Has there been a wild animal attack? Should we get ourselves to safety?
We lay our cards on the table and, running, follow the local who leads us to where we need to be. The light of our flashlights dances over the ground and, as we slow down, we all shine our light towards the same thing: on the ground lies one of the locals groaning in pain, shouting and screaming as if his life depends on it.
'Doctor!' his comrade calls out again, pointing to the man's crotch. I take a few steps closer, lean over the man, and immediately see what has happened. The poor guy fell on a stick about three feet long, and now it's sticking right through his scrotum.
'You guys need to see a doctor,' I say to one of the other locals, who have all gathered around their unfortunate friend. But they immediately shake their heads; that's too far away. It's also pitch black, it has rained, and the roads are bad.
'No,' someone else agrees. 'The doctor has to do it!' His finger points in my direction.
I hesitate, because my patients are actually animals, not humans. Technically speaking, humans are also a species of animal like all others, but a species of animal I have not studied.
'Please,' I hear from the ground, while the man moans and grabs my arm. I can't leave that poor man to his fate.
'Stay here,' I say, unlikely as it was that he would walk away in his condition. I hurry to the research station to get my equipment, then run back. I put on my gloves and disinfect my equipment like I would to carry out a procedure on any of my animals. I would never perform general anesthesia on a human, but I can administer local anesthesia.
'This may sting for a moment,' I warn.
'Oh no,' the young man moans. The whole team is gathered around

us, some are laughing, others look shocked. I try to remain calm, even though it's not easy with this, to me, unusual patient. I cut the stick as close to the wound as possible and then remove it as gently as I can.

'Stay still,' I say calmly, even though I have the impression the guy doesn't even dare to move.

'I will have to feel the wound for a moment.'

With my finger, I feel inside the scrotum to make sure the testicles have not been hit. And that's not the case.

'Everything is fine,' I say.

I disinfect and clean up the wound, and then have to sew up the scrotum.

I take a deep breath. A scrotum is a scrotum, whether it belongs to a human or an animal. Still, it does feel weird to do it with a human this time.

Finally, I can reassure the young man.

'I can give you painkillers and antibiotics,' I say. 'I have them in my suitcase.'

'Thank you,' he mumbles, completely confused.

'Don't worry,' I say. 'I knew what I was doing. I have performed castrations on animals before.' I laugh and wonder if that information would actually reassure him.

'But,' I continue, 'I must say, this is the first time I've left the balls in.'

2013-2022: Pairi Daiza, Belgium

I was working in Qatar when the owner of Pairi Daiza asked me if I wanted to come work for him. For the first time, two pandas would be coming to this Belgian zoo and they were looking for a veterinarian with zoo experience to oversee that project.

I had to think long and hard about that request. From experience, I knew that a change in job not only had implications for me, but also for my family. We were settled in Qatar and suddenly Belgium was an option again. It made us think, and that's when we realized: if we didn't return to Belgium now, we might never do it again.

So off we went.

At the time, I didn't really know what my job would entail. Though I did suspect that it would be more than just taking care of two pandas. Much more, as it quickly became apparent. I not only became the head veterinarian, but I would also be leading the zoological department. This meant that all the keepers would fall under my responsibility, along with animal-related matters, collection planning, assisting in the development of new enclosures, nutrition, animal transport, and contacts with other zoos. It was a steep learning curve, but one I followed with great pleasure.

During those nine years in Pairi Daiza, I had a top team of dedicated keepers and the best assistant anyone could imagine: Vanessa. She often knew what I needed before I did, and supported me through thick and thin.

Together, we have carried out some wonderful projects and often made the impossible possible.
For our family, returning to Belgium turned out to be an excellent move. Marie started playing music more again, and still plays in various orchestras today. The children quickly found their way at school with new friends. And to go full circle: all three children ride ponies, just like their dad used to do.

18. Pandamania

I'm nervous as I am being guided through the panda base in Dujiangyan, China, to the enclosures where I will meet pandas Hao Hao and Xing Hui for the first time. The handheld camera I received from a Flemish television channel to film everything is still in the bag I carry over my shoulder.

"There is Xing Hui,' I'm told, while a panda lying on its back in the grass is pointed to.

'And there's Hao Hao, the female.' She is leisurely leaning against a tree, nibbling on a bamboo stick. Both pandas are not impressed by our presence, although the opposite is certainly true.

I take out my handheld camera and aim it at the two animals looking at us with big eyes in adjacent enclosures. I catch myself smiling the whole time and I really realize now: these are such special animals. The giant panda has become the symbol of endangered species. There are only about 1600 individuals left, in a small part of China, Sichuan. Some pandas are kept in zoos worldwide, and Pairi Daiza will be one of them. I have the huge responsibility to manage that move smoothly.

'Are you impressed?' asks my Chinese colleague.

'Immensely,' I nod.

The two weeks in China give me the time to get to know the pandas personally, because each individual has its own character. I will help the keepers every day and learn, among other things, which bamboo they like, how much they eat and poop, because that is also important, and how panda cake is made. Panda cake is a source of extra energy and proteins for the pandas, and is made according to a secret recipe that zoos only get when they receive the pandas from China. In addition, I will also receive extra lessons in 'panda medicine' to learn how to recognize and treat possible diseases in pandas. I have two busy weeks ahead of me, but I'm really looking forward to it.

Somewhere halfway through those two weeks, I speak to Marie on the phone.
'There's a real pandamania going on here,' she says laughing. 'There's a huge hype about those pandas in the media right now. Every day something's published about them in the news, and there are even journalists camping at the children's school! They want to interview them about their dad and the pandas.'
'What?' I say, surprised.
'Yes!'
'I'll take care of it,' I say quickly. Marie's update surprises me, because I had no idea this story would take on such proportions in Belgium.
'Tim...' Marie says, sounding suddenly more serious. 'This is very special. You do realize that, right?'
I nod. 'I do now.'
The fact that this is such a big deal, however, doesn't intimidate me. On the contrary. It makes me even more excited about the adventure, and the tension rises even more the next day when the Belgian press also shows up in China, with teams for various TV channels. I talk to all of them, explaining each time what the departure here and the arrival in Belgium means for all the parties involved. Hao Hao and Xing Hui are not simply being bought or gifted by China. The Chinese government is only lending them to Belgium for fifteen years, as part of a breeding program. It's the first time China has made pandas available for such a long period of time.
The two weeks in China fly by, and during the farewell party I am completely blown away. And I'm not the only one: in the meantime, a whole Belgian delegation has also arrived, including the Belgian ambassador of China and the owner of Pairi Daiza. It's customary for China to celebrate the new homeland of the pandas, so for Belgium they have brought in Smurfs. The party will be a magnificent spectacle and it moves me when even school children perform to bid farewell to the pandas. During the festivities, far away from the noise and dancing, Hao Hao and Xing Hui are calmly loaded into the crates by the specialized keepers. Their two regular keepers don't leave their side, but I don't want to miss this crucial first phase

of the transportation process myself, either. I don't want anything to go wrong while I'm in charge. As often as I can, I check with my Chinese colleagues to see if everything is still okay, which seems to me to be the case.

After the ceremony, the pandas are placed in transparent boxes in the truck for the actual departure. When one of the keepers and the regular veterinarian of the pandas accompany me during the truck ride to the airport, Mr. Wu reassures me.

'You know...', he says. 'These are such calm animals. They adapt very quickly. For them, there is actually no difference between the truck ride they are used to and airplane transport.'

Together we drive for just over an hour to the airport and then the journey home can really begin, after a celebration is held at the airport by DHL, the transport company that will be operating a so-called panda flight for the first time.

I quickly take a photo of that airplane with my cell phone, which is painted with a huge panda logo designed by Marie herself.

I immediately forward the photo to her. 'Not only a talented musician, but also a talented artist,' I add with a wink, but I do mean it. The fact that she's also involved in the project that is changing our lives in a way is remarkable.

It's only when I look at that photo on my phone once more that I notice how much commotion there is again. The plane is surrounded by several TV crews and all cameras are focused on the pandas, who are being driven towards the plane on an airport trolley.

The pandas are loaded onto the plane with the utmost care. The cargo pallets are first rolled onto a lift in front of the plane, and then the pandas are lifted up, one by one, and rolled in through the large open aircraft door, where they are secured for the flight.

When they're all set, we can also get on board. I let my colleagues, the Chinese veterinarian, and the keeper go first. Then I get in.

This transport plane is special because there are only four seats and the rest of the cargo is empty, except for those two boxes with Hao Hao and Xing Hui. And a box with extra bamboo for the flight and the first days in Belgium.

We regularly approach Hao Hao and Xing Hui and observe them. 'And?' my colleagues keep asking. 'What do you think?' But the pandas are behaving exemplarily.
'I have veterinary supplies and medication with me,' I say. 'But it doesn't look like I'll need them.'
I feed the pandas some more bamboo shoots, and when we make a stopover in Bahrain they get panda cake.
'In my opinion, Hao Hao seems a bit nervous,' I remark to the keeper. He reassures me again, but promises to keep an eye on them with me. 'This is still the same truck ride for her,' he winks.
The flight goes smoothly, and faster than I expected. The landing is initiated with a few words from the airport control tower in Zaventem that will always stay with me:
'We cleared the whole airspace. You can enter with your precious cargo.'
I breathe a sigh of relief. We made it.
When the wheels of the airplane touch the ground, I eagerly look out the window. I only notice the welcoming committee when we come to a stop. The Belgian delegation, including Prime Minister Elio di Rupo and Minister of the Interior Alexander De Croo, is already waiting for us. And they're accompanied by about a hundred journalists. The local elementary school is also present, with all the children waving panda flags.
'The world is watching,' I say to my colleagues, surprised. They laugh as if it's not news to them. The arrival is a real media event, I realize once again. But now I see it with my own eyes.
On the runway, Hao Hao and Xing Hui are being shown to the audience and the press for the first time. The transparent cages were made opaque with panels featuring Smurfs, which were removed at the crucial moment. While the crowd is mesmerized by the two giant pandas, they seem hardly impressed at all. That reassures me. Before the final stage begins, we listen to a speech from Prime Minister Di Rupo.
'Di Rupo has my panda teddy bear in his hands,' I quickly send to Marie, with a smiling face. I bought that teddy bear a few days earli-

er at a local market in Chengdu and thought it would be nice to give it as a gift to the prime minister. I didn't expect him to give a speech with it. Later, this photo would go viral worldwide with the accompanying text: 'Belgian prime minister loves pandas.'

'The arrival of the pandas is very important for our country,' he says during his speech. 'Not only for the relations between China and Belgium, but also for the Belgian economy.'

People talk, listen, applaud, and then we can hit the road again. Finally.

Under police escort, with officers riding motorbikes ('swans'), and with a helicopter from Belgian commercial television channel VTM above us, and a motorcycle from French radio station RTL next to the truck, the journey continues to Pairi Daiza, our final destination. I almost can't believe my eyes, because even on the way people are waving next to the road, and a crowd of people is waiting for us at the zoo. Well, they are mainly waiting for the pandas. The zoo itself is currently still closed for the winter break, but opens today for all staff and family members, as well as those of DHL. Even my children are present with their class to do a little dance during the arrival party, which I arranged with the school. It also becomes a real family event for us, although I will miss most of that party because we will be unloading the pandas backstage while it's going on.

Our truck is trying to make its way through the sea of people to disappear into the backstage. The Belgian keepers are eagerly waiting to catch a first glimpse of the pandas. I stick up my thumb as we pull in. The whole team is ready with a forklift and pallet jack, and when the truck doors swing open, everyone springs into action.

Xing Hui is carefully unloaded and taken to his new enclosure first. The crate is placed against an interior door and strapped in securely to make it's safe to let him out. Fresh bamboo is placed in his enclosure and then we open the door. Very cautiously but curiously, he walks step by step out of his transport crate and starts to smell his new enclosure. He quickly settles in a corner and pulls some bamboo towards him to eat. The Belgian keepers and I get goosebumps when we see this, but we can't stay too long, because Hao Hao still needs to go to her new enclosure. We repeat the entire procedure and Hao Hao also emerges from her crate. She's a bit more active, but soon also starts to eat.

What a rush... After months of planning and preparation, our pandas have finally arrived.

'The pandas are okay,' I text my boss, who is at the ceremony, so he knows everything is fine.

The hours and even days after arrival, I'm just swept along with everything. I go from the pandas to the press and back again, all with some serious real jet lag. The first days are the most stressful days for the pandas. For example, they refuse to eat bamboo if it does not come from China, and our supply of Chinese bamboo is slowly running out. Only when they put aside their culinary preferences after a few days and start eating European bamboo, can I really enjoy it. Finally, I am at ease, because the pandas are also at ease.

The initial pandamania has subsided among the general public, but for me, the arrival of those pandas has meant and changed so much. Hao Hao and Xing Hui are not just pandas to me, they are a turning point in my professional life, as will become clear later.

19. Mouth-to-trunk ventilation

'There! A fetus! She's pregnant!' On the ultrasound, I see a small blob in the uterus of elephant Aye Chan May. I'm very impressed, just like the keepers standing next to me. I started this ultrasound with a lot of hope, but I actually didn't dare to think I would see signs of a pregnancy. Aye Chan May was successfully inseminated by our breeding male Po Chin 60 days ago, that much is clear now! Aye Chan May came to us in Pairi Daiza from Cologne Zoo because she didn't fit in with the group there. Elephants live in a matriarchal family group, led by the matriarch and her daughters and granddaughters. The bull elephants, or male elephants, leave the group after a few years. Aye Chan May was not related to the matriarch and other elephants, so she didn't really feel at home in that group. Here she has found her place in the elephant group, and now her position will only become stronger because an elephant that is pregnant is very important to the group.

This pregnancy is immediately the start of the whole journey to birth.

'Fantastic,' I whisper. 'I will start drafting a protocol right away.'

For each pregnant elephant, an individual protocol is drawn up, tailored to the needs of the particular animal. The protocol contains guidelines on blood sampling before birth to monitor the delivery properly, the timing of calcium administration to provide extra calcium when the calf's bony skeleton starts growing rapidly, any medication that should be available, and what to do if something goes wrong.

I also begin to count now: an elephant carries for 21 months, which is about 635 days. If we start counting from Aye Chan May's last mating date, we end up with the birth some time in July.

As soon as the pregnancy is confirmed, the keepers and I monitor Aye Chan May closely. The keepers pamper her even more, but also pay attention to how she is received in the group. It's important that the other elephants behave calmly around her, so that the pregnancy can continue without any stress. About two months before delivery, I start taking regular blood samples. First weekly, then every two days, until finally taking blood daily in the last two weeks before the due date. We monitor the progesterone levels because this is a very reliable way to predict labor in elephants. Progesterone is the pregnancy hormone and maintains the pregnancy, so these levels are very high throughout the pregnancy. When these start to decrease, the delivery is near and when the value falls below 3 mmol/ 34 oz, our elephant will give birth within 48 to 72 hours. We also regularly check the calcium level to see if there is enough calcium present for proper bone growth of the calf in the uterus, and later on for proper lactation.

'Strange,' I say as I review the results of her blood test. The progesterone level is actually low, lower than expected for sure. Her level makes me doubt if everything is okay with the pregnancy.

Throughout Aye Chan May's pregnancy, the level remains around that low point, so I assume that this may be normal for her, as there are always individual differences between animals. But still, it's strange compared to previous pregnancies I have supervised. Together with the head keeper, I make the decision to take her out of the group for the delivery. Aye Chan May just prefers to be alone sometimes and with those 'weird' progesterone levels, I'd rather not take any risks.

An elephant usually gives birth in the herd. In it, everyone has a role as an aunt, brother or sister, niece or nephew. It is very important for everyone in the group to experience the birth, because they learn from it as a group. As soon as an elephant gets contractions and starts to push, the group will stand around the mother. When the calf is finally born, all hell breaks loose. All the elephants then start to trumpet and make sounds, which cuts me to the bone. Every time the hairs on my arms stand up and I get chills. The joy is ecstatic. It's not just the birth, but also the dynamics of the elephant group that is so impressive. All those elephants walking back and forth with their massive legs and bulky bodies, without trampling that little calf. It may seem threatening at times, to outsiders, when the mother turns her head and bends over the calf, as if she wants to headbutt it, but she does that because her eyes are positioned sideways and otherwise can't see her calf. The way the mother tries to activate her calf and encourage it to stand up may also seem aggressive, but it's not. When the calf finally stands up and starts drinking, we consider it a success. And it's an unforgettable experience for everyone who witnesses it, because there are few things more impressive.

'She's quite new to the group,' I explain to the team. 'It's also possible that there will be problems with the calf. We'll monitor and take care of her as best as we can.'

The whole team agrees. Because every elephant is different and experiences pregnancy differently, we have no choice but to wait and see if everything is okay until the moment she gives birth.

A few days later, I take an ultrasound of Aye Chan May, because the progesterone level has dropped even further, which means that the delivery is imminent. So I want to know if the cervix is already starting to open, so that the calf can descend, or rather in the case of an elephant, come up, since the calf is located at the bottom of the abdomen and the birth canal is all the way at the top.

I let the team know: 'It's time'. 'Aye Chan May is dilating, so it won't take much longer now.'

At that moment, it feels like we are on some kind of team retreat. The following two nights we will actually stay on site, so we can monitor everything and intervene immediately if necessary. Those days and nights of being on call mean a lot to us and create a sense of togetherness.

Sometime halfway through the second night, one of the keepers announces,

'It's going to happen.' Immediately, we all gather around the TV screen in the kitchen. We don't want to disturb her during this intimate moment.

He might be right.

Aye Chan May is pacing restlessly, she's clearly struggling. She whips her tail back and forth, occasionally crossing her hind legs and pushing her head against the wall, indicating that she is having contractions and maybe even the urge to push.

'Almost there,' I say softly. Her keepers nod. Everyone keeps their gaze fixed on the impressive animal. It's night, but no one feels tired. There is too much adrenaline for that. I try to keep my nerves under control, but I'm still worried. What if something's wrong...

While Aye Chan May takes a few steps forward and backward in her box, I try to take in the moment. I see one keeper nervously clenching and relaxing his fists, and another constantly holding his hand in front of his mouth. I try to remain calm.

As a veterinarian, I often have to intervene actively, but there are also moments when I just have to stand by and watch. Like now. My presence would otherwise disrupt the normal course of events. The natural order decided that every animal should be able to give birth independently, so that is always our starting point.

Aye Chan May is getting more restless, slightly bending her hind legs, we see a bump appearing under her tail, and with one final push, the calf falls between her hind legs to the ground.

We all run downstairs to her enclosure.

The elephants in the nearby enclosure start trumpeting, but soon it becomes quiet. Unpleasantly quiet. No more stomping of other elephants, no more trumpeting. Even we dare not say anything. We wait and see, but the calf remains motionless on the ground.

Aye Chan May sniffs her calf with her trunk, but she still can't get it to move.

'We need to go inside,' I say, signaling to the keepers to gather all our equipment. The keepers lead me into the enclosure because they are familiar with Aye Chan May. I don't know her that well, so maybe she would see me as an intruder and feel threatened, especially now. It's a small space and she could easily trample us. I cautiously step into the enclosure, but I immediately notice that she is tolerating me. Would she realize that her calf is in danger? I wonder, although I don't want to or can't even imagine being in her shoes.

I kneel next to the calf and see that it is not breathing. I am overwhelmed by panic, but I also realize that I need to respond quickly.
I place my mouth at the end of the trunk and blow into it to start mouth-to-trunk resuscitation.

All eyes are fixed on me, but I try to shut out everything around me. I want only one thing: to save that calf.
I turn my head and take a deep breath, then once again breathe into the elephant.
'Yes!' I hear from behind me.
The baby elephant starts to breathe and move around. The trunk moves around uncontrollably and the legs move. I now examine the elephant further, looking into its eyes and immediately notice that the pupils are dilated, a condition known as mydriasis. The little one stares at me with a glassy look. We try to help the little elephant stand up straight, but it keeps collapsing. We work on the calf all night, while also regularly milking Aye Chan May to get the milk production going. She just stands there. Restless one moment, composed and waiting the next.
Once again, I put myself in her position. How much does she realize? I always try to be careful with anthropomorphism, attributing human characteristics to animals. Especially as a zoo, we're very aware of regular visitors who think they can establish a bond with a specific animal. No one should forget that these are still wild animals, to which you cannot simply attribute human characteristics or emotions. And yet. Yet here and now, I would venture to think that Aye Chan May is intelligent enough to realize that we are trying to save her young, as if she knows it's in danger.
'We'll wait for the morning,' I finally decide. 'If there is no improve-

ment... I fear brain damage.'
Everyone nods dejectedly. I, too, feel dejected.
The next day it turns out that there is no improvement. The baby elephant remains immobile and unresponsive, confirming my suspicions. Different neurological examinations do not bode well. There is no proprioception, meaning he does not straighten his feet when we block them. When we shine a light into the pupil, it does not get smaller, so the pupillary reflex is negative. There is indeed brain damage, and euthanasia is the only possible solution.
'We let Aye Chan May say goodbye to her calf,' I say, after which I prepare everything for the euthanasia and post-mortem of the calf. I call the Faculty of Veterinary Medicine in Ghent to ask if I can come with the calf to perform the autopsy together, and they confirm that it's possible. I hate it, but it's the only option. The best option.
Aye Chan May sniffs her calf with her trunk, but doesn't nudge it to get it move. I again get the feeling that she knows what's going on. In normal circumstances, the whole group would mourn the loss and the farewell would last for days. But Aye Chan May seems ready.
'Does she need to leave?' the keeper asks when he notices I'm ready.
'Let her stay,' I tell him. 'That's better for her.'
With a catheter in the ear, I administer the lethal injection to the elephant calf. The glassy look quickly becomes sleepy and eventually the little elephant closes its eyes, forever. This hurts me more than I thought it would, because elephants are my favorite animals and a baby elephant is just about the cutest thing you will ever see. The decision to put this little creature to sleep hits hard.
Aye Chan May lets it all happen, she's not even uneasy.
When the baby elephant has been euthanized, I look at Aye Chan May.
'She can rejoin the group, I think,' I say to the keeper.
The devastation within the team is huge. I can't help but feel this with them. This is in no way like how a normal birth occurs. This isn't how it should be. But it's just how it is this time.
The small, lifeless elephant is loaded into the car and I drive it to the Faculty of Veterinary Medicine in Merelbeke.

An autopsy reveals that the elephant indeed has a brain abnormality. Only the cerebellum is present, no cerebrum at all. Where the cerebrum should be, the cavity is filled with fluid, a condition known as hydrocephalus. The cerebellum is the reptilian brain and is responsible for breathing and heart rate. That explains why the elephant calf was viable, but otherwise non-functional.

It's also the reason, I realize now, why that progesterone level was always so low.

Could we have done something if we had known in advance? No. Even then, Aye Chan May would have had to carry the baby to term to know the extent of the damage and whether or not the calf would be viable. It was just bad luck and we will never truly know the real reason why it went wrong. There may have been a herpes infection in the uterus. That's known to lead to problems during pregnancy in other animal species, and elephant herpes is also a known issue in young calves, so who knows.

Two years later, Aye Chan May is pregnant again. Those 21 long months are a trial for everyone, as it is difficult to have faith after the loss of that little one. Only after the birth, when it becomes clear that the mother and her calf, Malee, are healthy, does that ecstatic joy return.

20. She's in heat

Yawning, I look at the time on my phone. It is 6pm local time, Australian time. I'm too tired to count back to Belgian time; that's how jet-lagged I am. It's my third day in Australia, where I'll be having koala training for a month, as koalas will soon be coming to Pairi Daiza. The day is almost over and I'm already looking forward to simply relaxing on the couch. My phone suddenly vibrates in my hand: incoming call from Tania. She's one of the permanent keepers of our pandas Hao Hao and Xing Hui at Pairi Daiza.

'I think Hao Hao is going in heat,' she says.

I'm wide awake now. If this is true, it means she's ready for fertilization and a possible pregnancy!

Reproduction in giant pandas is a big mystery for several reasons. Giant pandas are only fertile for a short period of time, 12 to 24 hours per year. And even then, determining that moment of fertility is a challenge. Diagnosing a pregnancy after fertilization is also very difficult. A panda pregnancy lasts about 136 days or around four and a half months, divided into two different phases. The first phase is known as the phase of 'delayed implantation', where the fertilized egg divides a few times and then floats around in the uterus. This phase lasts about three and a half months. After this stage, the embryo finally attaches to the uterine wall and the second phase begins, the pregnancy period of about 42 days.

Since the arrival of Hao Hao and Xing Hui, we had been looking for a lab and researcher who could monitor Hao Hao's heat and pregnancy. Through many detours and trial and error, we ended up with Jella, a scientist from the Faculty of Veterinary Medicine at Ghent University who is happy to help develop a research method to predict when a giant panda is in heat, pregnant, and when she will give birth.

'She eats noticeably less and displays more aggressive behavior than

usual,' Tania continues.
'Has Jella confirmed it yet?' I ask. Without that confirmation we'll have to keep guessing, I'm afraid.
'She's working on it. I've sent the urine samples to her lab. I'll keep you posted.' That same evening I receive another phone call, this time from Jella.
'I think you should return to Belgium. It's time; ovulation is approaching.'
I can't believe my ears. I immediately book the first possible flight to Belgium, and when I arrive there I go straight to the Faculty of Veterinary Medicine to consult with the reproduction team. They normally work with small to medium-sized pets and therefore have the right equipment for insemination. If we were to actually get that far. The anesthesiology department will be contacted and the dean of the faculty will be informed, because this is significant. A team of Chinese specialists is also on its way. Everything and everyone is being prepared, and hour after hour, conversation after conversation, the tension rises. The tension that helps me survive the deadly fatigue of my second jet lag in just over a week.
Once we were able to schedule a first meeting with everyone, a Chinese specialist takes the floor.
'The first option is always natural fertilization. Only when that fails, we will proceed with artificial insemination.'
I nod. Everyone nods. The man is so authoritative that we trust him blindly.
'Our technique is simple,' he continues. 'We take a bamboo stick and push it against the panda's backside. If the panda responds by walking backwards and 'neighing', we have the right moment.
There's chuckling. So many specialists in one room, so much knowledge and techniques. And a bamboo stick will tell us when it's time. Nature is amazing.
'At the same time, the hormone specialist will always perform a urine test to determine the moment of ovulation as accurately as possible.'
First, the estrogen level should rise, then ovulation follows and the estrogen level suddenly drops. This decline gives us 12 hours to have

a successful fertilization. From then on, playtime is over. All the research, all the thinking, all the contacts... Everything has led to this moment.

'Not yet,' says the hormone specialist. More than once.

'Not yet,' every time the estrogen level has not yet dropped.

Meanwhile, Hao Hao is, of course, being closely monitored and poked with that bamboo stick. Her behavior is clearly changing. She urinates more, walks around more, and often seeks cooling in the water because her vulva is red, warm and swollen. She also vocalizes often, but we haven't heard that typical neighing yet. Her tail is already going up occasionally when we touch her vulva with the bamboo stick, but she is not walking backwards yet.

Two days after the start of the intensive monitoring, she finally responds positively to the nudging by clearly neighing and walking backwards, as if she is offering herself for mating. The hormone specialist also brings positive news.

'Yes. This is it. The estrogen dropped.'

Now that we have determined the moment of ovulation, we can prepare for the fertilization.

'We will first try the natural way,' the Chinese specialist repeats. We take Xing Hui to Hao Hao's enclosure. When he enters the backstage area, he immediately smells the hormones of the female.

'That's a good sign,' I mutter.

Hao Hao is in the adjacent enclosure and immediately notices Xing Hui. They first sniff each other through the bars until Hao Hao turns around and raises her tail. Xing Hui clearly finds it all quite interesting and seizes his chance, but Hao Hao turns around and becomes aggressive every time he gets closer. She reaches out to him through the bars and attacks.

The Chinese specialist intervenes. 'We're calling it quits,' he says. 'The risk is too great and Xing Hui is getting scared.'

Xing Hui is taken back to his enclosure, the door closes behind him as he walks away, and we move on to our plan B: artificial insemination. We will perform this procedure twice. 6 hours after ovulation, which Jella was able to determine exactly, and a second time 12 hours later. Immediately, I call the reproduction specialists in Ghent to jump in their car for the insemination. When everyone has arrived, you can already feel the excitement. We're going to do something special tonight. There are very few pandas outside of China, so very few Western veterinarians ever get to experience this. Nervous, everyone sets up their equipment so we can start.

It's my turn first. I prepare a tranquilizer dart and shoot it into Xing Hui's buttocks with the rifle, causing him to fall asleep shortly after. 'Come on,' I say, when I'm sure he's out. Together with the keeper and an anesthesiologist from Ghent, I enter his cage. I open his mouth and insert a tube into his throat so he can be ventilated. He's then placed on a stretcher and transferred to the panda hospital. In all zoos worldwide, each panda enclosure has its own panda hospital on site, where only pandas are allowed to be treated. In our case, the hospital is located in the panda cave of the female Hao Hao. All the materials and equipment necessary to treat pandas are available at all times, if required.

Once Xing Hui is lying on the examination table, I switch to gas anesthesia and shave a small piece of hair on his forearm to insert a catheter. It is always important during anesthesia to have access to a blood vessel, in case you need to administer medication quickly. Everyone in the team, a dozen specialists in various fields, is now doing their thing, in utmost concentration. Xing Hui will receive an ultrasound of the heart, lungs and abdominal organs, and I will monitor the anesthesia. An ultrasound of the testicles is also performed to measure them, after which it is time for electroejaculation.

'The probe is being inserted,' is announced. A long rod is inserted rectally into Xing Hui, so that electric stimuli can be administered near his prostate. That needs to be done several times until Xing Hui ejaculates and the sperm can be collected.

'Success!' I hear.

I laugh. On the one hand relief, on the other hand the thought that Xing Hui probably imagined that fertilization differently.

'Check semen.' The next step. Immediately, the sperm is examined microscopically to check the sperm's mobility, how the sperm cells

move, the ratio of living sperm cells to dead ones, and the quality.
'Repetition of the procedure.'
Eventually, three ejaculates are successfully collected, which after dilution and a check can be used for inseminating Hao Hao.
'Done.'
Everyone can breathe a sigh of relief again. The first hurdle is over.
Xing Hui is transported back to his enclosure, and there I administer an injection to help him wake up. All the while, he is under the supervision of his keeper.
Then it's time for the next phase. Once again, I prepare an anesthetic that I will shoot into Hao Hao's buttock. She is transported to the hospital in the same way, where she is constantly monitored and receives an ultrasound of the uterus and ovaries.
'Ovulation has occurred on one side. Not yet on the other. So we can proceed.'
With the help of a vaginal speculum, an insemination pipette is inserted so that the insemination can take place in the cervix.
It's wonderful to see: on the ultrasound images, you can follow live how the sperm is injected and finds its way.
'That's it, we can't do more than that,' concludes the Chinese specialist. I clap and the rest follows. We're not there yet, but we're on the right track. Hao Hao is brought back to her enclosure and also receives an injection to wake up. This process will be repeated twelve hours later, so we can do a total of two inseminations.
After Hao Hao was returned to her enclosure following the second anesthesia and insemination, I receive a text message from the director of the zoo.
'Great job! You're expected at the press conference.' I read.
I accompany my Chinese colleague to the room where the press conference will take place and along the way ask him the question that perhaps everyone is wondering now.
'How likely is it that it worked? How likely is it that Hao Hao will be pregnant soon?'
The Chinese specialist looks at me with a big smile.
'90 percent,' he says, brimming with confidence.

The confidence is admirable, but I am more cautious myself. We must not be too hasty, give people false hope, or overestimate ourselves. Furthermore, a waiting period of 135 days will now follow, only then will we know for sure if it has been successful.
'That's great,' I say. 'But I'm afraid we won't be able to say that to the press in a moment.'
'I beg to differ,' he kindly replies. 'The conditions were good. This worked.'
'Let's wait and see,' I suggest, hoping that his answer at the press conference will be a bit more moderate. Because that question is asked.
'How likely is it that Hao Hao will be pregnant soon?' one of the journalists asks.
The Chinese specialist first looks at me and then at the journalist, with a broad smile.
'30 percent.'

21. A small, pink sausage

Quickly making an ultrasound to check if Hao Hao is pregnant is not an option for us. A panda may look cute, but it is and remains a wild animal. Especially our Hao Hao who has made it clear multiple times before she's not interested in a cold probe on her belly. It wouldn't be wise to enter her panda enclosure to perform an ultrasound. So we need to do it in a different way. The keepers observe Hao Hao constantly, looking for small or big changes in her behaviors, and her urine is also collected and examined for various hormones on a daily basis. In a panda, we usually count 140 days between fertilization and birth. We also use that calculation for Hao Hao to pinpoint an estimated date, but it doesn't tell us if she is pregnant or not. If we were to only look at progesterone, the pregnancy hormone, like with most other animals, a positive result from that test does not provide certainty with pandas. Pandas can actually experience pseudopregnancy, and the progesterone level in pandas increases both during pregnancy and pseudopregnancy. So when we want to make a distinction between the two, we need to look at different hormones and not just progesterone.

That's a complicated task, but everything is closely monitored by our hormone specialist Jella. If we do this correctly, we will know whether Hao Hao is actually pregnant approximately 24 days before the expected birth.

I get a phone call.

'Jella UGent' I read on the screen.

'Hello, Tim. The analyses look good. PGFM has increased and remains high. The estrogens have also slightly increased. I believe Hao Hao is indeed pregnant.'

Happiness, stress, anxiety, disbelief; I feel it all as I hang up the phone. I take a deep breath, then call China to have the specialists come and start the final preparations for our, hopefully, first panda baby.

‘We did it,’ Jella says. She proudly waves the papers showing the results of the urine test. ‘There has been an LH peak, which means we are 24 to 48 hours away from delivery.’
‘Incredible.’ Tanja, one of Hao Hao's regular keepers, covers her mouth with her hand, expressing what we are all thinking. It's unbelievable. This is what we have worked towards for so long, this is what we have tried so hard for.
From then on, the established protocol goes into effect. The keepers know when to keep watch over Hao Hao, and I also remain on standby. This is definitely something I wouldn't want to miss for the world.
Hao Hao herself also feels that something is about to happen.
‘She's restless, do you see that?’ Tanja asks, as I watch the live camera footage from the panda enclosure with her at the observation room. Our Chinese specialist, Mr. Wu, goes away to quickly freshen up.
I nod. I don't know Hao Hao as well as Tanja, who works with her constantly, but I also see that her behavior is different than usual. Hao Hao is very restless and does not seem to know what to do with herself. Sometimes she curls herself up into a ball and remains motionless for minutes, while other times she lies on her back and pushes her feet against the wall. It goes on like this constantly, for hours on end.
'Wouldn't you like to rest a bit?' Tanja asks me. She must have noticed the yawn I was trying to suppress after all. It's the middle of the night now, but I can't possibly go to sleep. I don't want to miss my date with history here.
‘No way. We‘re going ride this out together, with Hao Hao.’
We both continue to stare at the monitor, lost in thought, until we are startled by a loud, sharp scream.
'Wow!' Tanja exclaims, and I too am immediately alert. Mr. Wu runs into the room.

Hao Hao also seems startled by the scream. She turns around to see where that scream came from, and then we see, together with her, the baby panda lying on the ground in front of her.

'Nooooo way, amazing!' Tanja cries out. Our three noses are almost glued to the monitor. The baby panda is nothing more than some kind of small, pink sausage. Naked and hairless. But it certainly makes enough noise. It cries and cries to get Hao Hao's attention. It does this instinctively. Pandas are equally likely to have a single cub as they are to have twins. When the birth of twins happens in the wild, one young will always die, because the mother cannot keep two young with her. Hence the loud screaming. The little one making the most noise probably has the strongest survival instinct and is therefore picked up and taken away in the mother's mouth, in search of food.

By now we're already watching in front of the enclosure, with tears of joy in our eyes.

Hao Hao leans towards the squealing, picks up the cub in her mouth and places it on her belly. The young one immediately searches for the nipples, looking for milk. Hao Hao looks visibly exhausted, lying there as if she literally and figuratively can't lift up a paw anymore. Mr. Wu wants to weigh and check the baby as soon as possible to see that everything is okay. So he prepares a stick which he generously coats with honey. Because Hao Hao is so exhausted, he can just enter the enclosure and hand her the stick so she can lick the honey off to get some energy. While Hao Hao indulges herself with the honey, Mr. Wu can milk her.

'We have 1.5 ounces,' he quickly says. 'That's enough for now.'

Meanwhile, Mr. Wei, the second Chinese specialist, has already taken the baby and placed it in the incubator set to a comfortable 98°F.

Tanja and I are now standing next to Mr. Wei, intently watching how he handles this small, wondrous creature.
'6 ounces,' he says. 'That's a good weight for a baby panda.'
Tanja and I look at each other with beaming smiles. We've read that baby pandas weigh between 2.5 and 7 ounces at birth, and our baby, at 6 ounces, is a chubby one.
'Baby boy,' he says afterwards.
It's a boy. We are ecstatic.
According to Chinese tradition, panda cubs are only given a name when they are 100 days old, during an official ceremony. Until then, he is known as 'Baby Boy'.
Now that we know his weight and sex, we prepare the first bottle. It's important that Baby Boy receives the first milk as soon as possible, because it's so rich in antibodies. The aim is for the young one to gain about 1.8 to 3.5 ounces each day. The weight of adult pandas corresponds to about a thousand times the birth weight. In a human, that would mean we would weigh 6,600 pounds. I am quite heavy, but I'm not quite there yet, thankfully.
Mr. Wei specializes in hand-rearing baby pandas; that is his sole task at the breeding center in China. Tanja will start training with him, so that she can prepare and give the bottle herself within a few days or weeks, if necessary, but for now we observe how he does it. A panda baby is so small and almost breakable that both Tanja and I are glad we have these specialists here to help us and to learn from them.
Hao Hao's job now is to regain her strength.
When that happens, mother and child will be reunited. Both will still be observed and monitored. At first, the cub will be taken from Hao Hao every day to be weighed and, if necessary, fed a little more. After that, it'll be taken every three to four days to check its weight. Hao Hao also needs to step on the scale regularly. Even her feces are collected and weighed every day. It's important for milk production that she eats enough. That's why we also give her panda cake, which is high in proteins, and bamboo shoots, which are much richer in carbohydrates or sugars.
Mother and cub are given 100 days to get used to each other and to

life in the panda enclosure. Only then will they be presented to the general public, with a grand naming ceremony with China's ambassador in Belgium, a Belgian minister and the entire Belgian press. By then, the cub will be a cute, furry little ball named Tian Bao, which means 'heavenly gift'.

The day Tian Bao was born, Belgium made headlines worldwide. I received a phone call that day from former colleagues in Brazil and Australia saying they saw me on TV. We can be proud that we succeeded. And we are, almost as if we were the proud parents.

22. The last male on earth

'Hello Thomas, what can I do for you?' Thomas is a very good friend and THE world specialist in wild animal reproduction. When he calls, something special is often about to happen.

'Do you remember when we collected semen in Dvur Kralove in the Czech Republic, from that northern white rhino that then went to Kenya?'

Of course I remember. This rhino is the last male rhino of his species, and there are only three females left.

'Meanwhile, we have developed a technique to perform ovum pick-up in rhinos and we would like to try this on one of your rhinos. It might be able to save this species.'

In horses, this technique of collecting eggs and fertilizing them in vitro has been around for much longer, and Thomas and his team have adapted and fine-tuned that technique in rhinos. We agree to administer hormones to one of our rhinos before their visit, so that extra eggs can grow and be collected.

Our rhino is of a different species, namely the southern white rhino. But once the technique is perfected, this species could serve as a surrogate mother for the northern white rhino. The sperm of the 'last male on earth' and the eggs of one of the three surviving females could then be fertilized in vitro and implanted in southern white rhino females, like ours. But first, the technique must be flawless.

That morning I prepare my anesthesia dart to first perform a standing sedation on Eleonore, the rhino. We want to keep general anesthesia as short as possible, so we try to perform all procedures we can on the standing animal first. The dart is shot behind the ears, where the skin is softest and thinnest. After about ten minutes, the rhino is leaning against the metal bars of the enclosure and I can walk inside to put a blindfold on her and put cotton wool in her ears so she experiences minimal external stimuli.

Thomas is performing a rectal ultrasound in the meantime, and is

very happy with the result.
'I count dozens of eggs in both ovaries,' he says somewhat excited.
I now administer a second injection into a blood vessel in the ear, putting the rhino under full anesthesia.
'Open up,' I say, and three people help me get the mouth open. I have to reach into her mouth with my arm to insert the tube directly into her windpipe. It takes a little while, because I have to go quite deep, but I eventually manage to intubate her. 'Got it,' I sigh. Now we can smoothly transition to gas anesthesia and continue monitoring the anesthesia.
Thomas inserts a self-developed tube into the rectum to which the ultrasound probe is connected. He's looking for the ovaries and keeps the tube in place there. The ultrasound visualizes the entire process. Through a small opening in the tube, a needle is inserted above the ovary. He then punctures through the wall of the rectum, right into the ovary, into the egg. A vacuum is created and the egg is sucked into the needle towards the vacuum device.
'Unbelievable,' I mutter. 'You can just see the black egg disappear and then the ovary turns white again.'
I've never seen this before and I immediately feel like this could be huge if it works. 'Egg by egg,' Thomas says with utmost concentration. And just like that, egg by egg, he first empties the left ovary and then the right one.
'We have everything,' he concludes after more than an hour's work. 'All eggs are safely stored.'
'It's your turn again, Tim.'
I nod and can wake Eleonore once more. After all the equipment and people have been removed from the enclosure, I administer an antibody in the bloodstream. A few minutes later, she calmly stands up again, like nothing had happened.
Suzanne, a colleague of Thomas, is meanwhile examining all the eggs under the microscope. The eggs containing a nucleus are preserved, as they can be used for in vitro fertilization.
'We have five,' she says. 'Five usable eggs.'
The eggs are sent to Italy by plane, to the specialist who developed in

vitro fertilization for horses. The technique he uses is called ICSI: intra-cytoplasmic sperm injection, where a single sperm cell is injected into an egg to develop into an embryo in a test tube.
A few weeks later, Thomas calls again.
'Tim, I have good news. We were able to create two embryos from Eleonore's eggs.'
'No way...' I say, surprised. I wouldn't have dared to hope for this.
'The embryos have been frozen. Hopefully we can implant them in rhinos soon, but that technique still needs further development.'

Thomas continues to elaborate, but my thoughts wander off. This is actually big. Huge. This is the first step to save the northern white rhino from extinction.

Not One More Vet

'An changed her profile picture: NOMV.'
'Frederik changed his profile picture: NOMV.'
I saw about ten more of these notifications.
The accompanying article was always the same as well: 'It's with great sadness and dismay that we have learned that our colleague has taken their own life...'
This time, it was a young veterinarian who had graduated from the Faculty of Veterinary Medicine in Ghent just a few years previously. He had decided he'd had enough.
NOMV! 'Not One More Vet' is a slogan I unfortunately come across a little too often among veterinary colleagues around the world, but with this colleague it really hit very close to home. Not that I knew the colleague in question, but it did affect me. Our oldest son is also studying veterinary medicine, so I unconsciously thought of him. It could be your child. The suicide rates among veterinarians are 2.5 to 3 times higher compared to other professions.
As an eight-year-old boy, I already wanted to become a veterinarian, the coolest profession in the world in my eyes. When the veterinarian, Jaak, came to visit us, I hung on his every word and wanted to know everything about the sick animal. I even got to ride with him once. He was clearly my superhero and way cooler than Superman or Batman. Now, many years later, he is the godfather of our youngest daughter, Laura-Marie, and still my hero.
When I went to college, I didn't hesitate for a second about my choice of study. I was determined to become

a veterinarian, just like Jaak. I passed my first year with distinction and the greatest feeling of satisfaction. I was on my way to becoming a veterinarian.

I enjoyed every minute of my studies, except for the exams. After six years of study, I was ready to enter the profession. When I think about this, I'm convinced that for most veterinary students, it goes like this: the love for animals, that absolute passion to be able to practice the most wonderful profession in the world, pushes everyone through those studies.

It's only after those six years that you realize how little you know, despite the massive amount of knowledge you have acquired during your studies. And then fear strikes you to the core.

'What should I do now?'

'The lives of those animals depend on me, but I still don't know how to treat them at all.'

'And the owners, what should I tell them?'

These are all thoughts that plague every young veterinarian. I was fortunate to further specialize at the Faculty of Veterinary Medicine and to have someone like Jaak by my side in the practice on weekends. That way, I wasn't alone in this. Many young colleagues that try on their own or don't have support are often easily discouraged. At the twenty-year reunion of our graduating class, it was striking how very few colleagues are actually working as practicing veterinarians. The dropout rate, especially in the first years, is extremely high. And that for people who all started their studies with the dream of becoming a veterinarian.

How is it possible that passionate veterinarians become so discouraged that they quit the profession, or worse, take their own lives?

I ask myself that question every time I see another message with #Notonemorevet. When I look at myself, I know why I became a veterinarian. I much prefer animals to most people. Animals are honest. If they like you, they want your attention. If they don't like you, they'll bite or kick you. That's clear, everyone knows where they stand. People, on the other hand, can sometimes be sneaky, deceitful, and dishonest. They smile to your face and can stab you in the back when you're not looking. I think veterinarians often have the same hope for the people around them as they do for their animals. So it hurts a lot when they are deceived, maybe more than for other people.

As veterinarians, we come into contact with the owners of our animals on a daily basis. Those owners have often already spoken with Dr. Google and therefore think they know in advance and better than the vet what needs to happen to their pet. This sometimes leads to long discussions when the vet has a different idea than that renowned Dr. Google. When pet owners are not satisfied, they often do not hesitate to leave negative and sometimes aggressive reviews on social media in order to damage the reputation of a veterinarian. You have to be very strong to ignore this and just continue as if nothing had happened.

Not too long ago, I received death threats via Facebook. In the zoo where I used to work, a gorilla killed a mangabey monkey in a play fight. This was filmed, and the footage immediately appeared on social media. The press jumped on it and I had to speak to the press as a veterinarian. Gorillas and mangabeys often live together in the wild as well as in zoos, and they frequently interact with each other. In zoos, mixed-species exhibits are very popular because this is a huge enrichment for all the animals concerned. This has been studied and is now being implemented as standard in all modern zoos, with the necessary safety measures, of course. But after that interview, some people apparently thought it was a good idea to send me open death threats. That hits home, I assure you. I was really devastated by that, even after twenty years of being a veterinarian. If something like this had happened at the beginning of my career, I would have found it very difficult to comprehend.

What is often not said out loud among veterinarians is that our profession is actually a very uncollegial profession. Animal versus human, remember. Every man for himself. Veterinarians sometimes speak negatively about colleagues to customers, hoping to retain that new customer. Customers are calling around for the cheapest vaccine or the cheapest sterilization, and veterinarians are playing along by working cheaper than their colleague a few miles away. The story of veterinarians racing to a cesarean and running each other off the road to be the first on the scene is not unfamiliar in our world. Young colleagues often have to work as false self-employed for a ridiculously low wage, long hours, day and often night, with those older and more experienced veterinarians. That's downright discouraging.

In England, I worked in a group practice as an employee with a good salary and colleagues who supported each other's success, because we were not competitors. Fortunately, there has been some progress in recent years, but we still have a long way to go in Belgium.

And last but not least, the current veterinary training is not adapted to the reality of the profession. By the time we graduate, we have a mountain of knowledge about animals, diseases, treatments, and even surgical techniques, but very little knowledge about working as a self-employed person and dealing with customers and colleagues - we are often also psychologists for the human primates in our practice.
If we want Not One More Vet, we all need to take a good look at ourselves. It starts with the training, where there should be more emphasis on the human aspect of our profession. Veterinarians should collaborate more and support each other; after all, we still have the best profession in the world. And the customer, you, readers of my book, when you come to the vet, know that we are also just humans who want to save your pet. At all costs, day and night, weekdays and holidays. Give us a smile, a pat on the back, a compliment. That small gesture could potentially save a life.

23. From hero to poacher

'Have you heard the news about Hurricane Maria?'
On the other end of the line is Martin, a good friend and founder of the Association for the Conservation of Threatened Parrots (ACTP), an organization dedicated to the conservation and protection of endangered parrots and their habitat.
I nod. Hurricane Maria, the fourth major hurricane of this year, has hit the volcanic island of Dominica in the Caribbean Sea with full force. In a news report, the island's prime minister announces that the island has 'lost all that money can buy'. There is utter destruction. An entire population has lost its home, families are suffering losses - it's terrible. But in addition to those human losses, the exceptional natural landscape, home to so many animals, has been devastated.
On the island of Dominica, there are several indigenous amazon parrots, including the endangered ara arausiaca, also known as the red-necked amazon, and the imperial amazon, a colorful parrot about 18 inches long. It's the emblem of Dominica, depicted on the flag.
'The government of Dominica contacted me because the entire habitat of the imperial amazon has been blown away. They now realize that, like the other islands in the Caribbean, they need to have a *safety net population* outside of Dominica. I have been asked to go there and collect some of the birds,' Martin continues.
'Wow,' I respond. That's not nothing. A safety net population is a type of reserve population that is established and conserved outside the natural habitat of the animals in question. If a hurricane comes through in the area of origin, like in this case, that reserve population is there to ensure that the species does not go completely extinct.
'Will you come with me?' Martin asks.
'Yes, definitely, but first I need to explain to Marie that I'm going to fly halfway around the world to save some parrots.'
The next day we're already on our way to Dominica on a chartered plane. There is a lot of turbulence that shakes us around in our seats.

It has already been a long journey, with a layover in Canada at -4°F and over 3 feet of snow, only to finally arrive in Saint Lucia under a blazing sun. From there, we will continue the next day on a final charter flight using a propeller plane. Jet engine aircrafts can no longer land in Dominica; the airport infrastructure has been completely destroyed by the hurricane. 'We,' that's Martin, a specialized avian veterinarian, an editor-in-chief of a magazine about parrots, and me. 'Shit...' I say, when I finally see the island appear as I look outside. From the air, we now witness the devastation.

The entire island has been reduced to one big, gray patch. The rain forest, which is normally a green oasis, has been completely destroyed. You can't even see where the trees used to be. It's utter chaos. Everything is gray. Dead.

'Are you okay?' Martin asks during the car ride to our hotel after landing. The hotel is located in one of the few places where the hurricane has been mild.
'Gosh…' I mutter. I'm not okay, actually. I feel tears burning in my eyes. It feels so unreal, so incredibly emotional to see this up close. I don't know what things would look like after a nuclear bomb, but I think this isn't too far off ... Nature can be so beautiful, but also so cruel.
It's early evening, and due to the power outage it will soon be pitch dark throughout the island. The government has agreed that we will take the parrots with us the next morning and fly them to Germany, to Martin's center.
Once we arrive at the hotel, things don't get much better. Several people are busy cleaning up the mess. Leaning against one of the walls, I see a stroller, a surfboard and a bike; everything is broken. Trash is everywhere, as if garbage bags had been tossed around for fun. There's trash under the fallen branches and around what remains of the standing trees.

We quietly make our way to our hotel room, carrying our equipment bag.

'How silly this looks,' I say as I take our net out of the equipment bag and wave it in the air.

Martin grabs the net from my hands and catches me with it.

'There you go, the first plump parrot has been caught.' For the first time, we laugh again and forget for a moment the devastation that surrounds us.

After a turbulent night, we start our rescue of the birds. The government has allowed us to take ten birds: two imperial amazons and eight red-necked amazons.

We load the transport crates into the trunk of our rental car and drive to a bird sanctuary in the central park in the middle of the city. The journey there seems like another ride through hell. It may sound strange, but it warms my heart to see those birds upon arrival. Their colors, their obliviousness to what has happened on their island... They bring some joy to a sad, sad situation.

Martin, veterinarian Marcellus, and I are making a plan to catch the birds as stress-free as possible. Marcellus enters the aviary with the net and with a quick swish he has already caught the first parrot. Under a deafening screech, he carefully takes it out of the net and together we quickly examine the parrot. We check the mouth for any yellow plaques, feel the chest to assess the body condition, and quickly inspect the feathers and legs. Everything seems fine and we put it in the transport box. We repeat this until all birds are safely stored in the dark box.

When we leave the building, we are thanked profusely by the keepers and by Thomas, the government official in charge.

'We can't thank you enough for saving these animals.' Thomas gives us the necessary official paperwork to export the animals, and we get into the car to drive back to the airport on what remains of the roads. A journey that normally takes half an hour now takes almost two.

It seems a bit strange to be thanked so much for the simple fact that we are doing our job, while we are now leaving them in ruins and chaos.

I am happy when we start the return journey to Berlin that evening, with the ten birds next to us on the empty seats, so we can observe them continuously on the plane.

'This is the shortest city trip I've ever taken,' Martin remarks sarcastically. I have to smile about it.

'Me too,' I agree. 'Me too…' It warms my heart to still be able to laugh with Martin about silly things every now and then, because otherwise this would hit even harder. It feels strange to leave the people in Dominica behind, without being able to do much more for them. But perhaps the most important thing at such a time is to do what you can. And taking care of those birds, which ultimately are also part of the island's identity, is what we can and will do.

On a layover in Canada to refuel, I'm relieved we have already made it this far. The parrots are calm and have already eaten and drunk. From here, straight to Berlin.

'Uh oh,' I hear Martin say before he gets out.

I see we're being met by two airport security agents, and as I follow a few feet behind Martin, I'm also waved over by one of them.

'Do you have permission to fly with those animals?' I hear them ask when I reach them.

'Of course,' Martin replies, immediately diving into his suitcase to show the necessary papers. He looks calm and composed, but I can feel my nerves racing through my body. I can already guess what happened: conservationists who are also working in Dominica must have seen us leave with the birds, and without knowing the full story assumed we came to steal them. We may have the permission of Dominica's government, but if nothing has been officially arranged and communicated to the CITES authorities, then we can claim whatever we want. CITES is the international legislation that regulates the export and import of endangered species, and has been adopted by most countries in the world. Without these papers, our endangered birds are not allowed to travel and we would have taken them illegally from their country of origin. Then we would indeed be considered poachers! Especially since we stayed on Dominica for such a short time. Load up and go! That's what it seems like right now. We have suddenly gone from hero to poacher...

'Could you follow us, please?' the men ask. Which we do. We are taken to a small office in the airport, where there are phone calls busily being made. Martin takes the lead as he is aware of the administration that has taken place and tries to resolve the issue. Which he manages to do. After a lot of bravado, back-and-forth phone calls and emails, all official documents appear to be in order.
'This is Dominica's statement that a collaboration has been signed stating that we will take care of the *safety net population*. This is a statement from the German government confirming the same.'
The misunderstanding is resolved and we can continue our flight to Berlin with the ten birds, and then drive to the center of the Association for the Conservation of Threatened Parrots by car.
The birds are still there years later and have successfully bred in captivity. Their *safety net population* is now a reality.

24. The World of the Cold

'This is Garik, the male. And that's Frosya, the female.'

In the tiny pool in front of me, two walruses are swimming in circles, almost in a stereotypical manner. Garik immediately stands out because of his short, straight tusks. Frosya is a small animal with a very rectangular and flat head, on which she has a number of spots or scratches. She seems like a rather shy animal. I notice her tusks are broken.

'Fine walruses,' concludes the veterinarian of the Utrish Marine Station near Anapa on the Russian coast of the Black Sea, not far from Crimea. She seems proud, but I get the feeling that we are here to save these animals and give them a better future. Because that's why I'm here: in Pairi Daiza, in The World of the Cold, there is a hypermodern and large walrus enclosure which already contains three females that have arrived from Valencia in Spain via Hamburg in Germany, but we still don't have a sexually mature breeding male for them. That's what I find here, in Russia. Garik and Frosya have been living together their whole lives, so we have decided to bring them both to Belgium. These two specimens were in the St. Petersburg aquarium, but it suddenly had to close. Then they were brought here to Utrish in a higgledy-piggledy manner with their trusted keepers, but clearly under suboptimal conditions.

'Are those tusks rinsed?' I immediately ask the veterinarian, who nods after translating my English into Russian.

'I'll show you later,' she confirms.

In preparation for this visit, I had already received a crash course in walrus zookeeping. A new addition to my RESUME, alongside that of truck driver. Because we are in the midst of the Covid crisis and Russia is no longer issuing visas, my presence must be justified. A visa is only granted for medical reasons or for truck drivers carrying out transportation. Since I have no immediate plans to have surgery in Russia, I have opted for the latter option.

This week, I will learn more ins and outs from the local keepers: what behaviors can the walruses exhibit, how can I teach them behaviors, how are they fed, and so on. It quickly becomes apparent that the behaviors of these two walruses are based on circus tricks. They can juggle, catch hoops, and give kisses, things we don't teach in the modern zoo. At our place, behaviors are mainly medically based, so the veterinarian can examine the animal without any stress. I also watch the veterinarian taking blood and rinsing the tusks each day. She shows me the disinfectant she uses. Everything is in Russian, so it needs to be translated for me. I have never heard of the agent and when I look it up, it also doesn't seem to exist in Europe. It's a remnant of the former Soviet period, and I silently decide that I will use a different disinfectant in Belgium, such as chlorhexidine.
'All the pus has to come out,' she remarks during a rinse, though I know that even without her explanation. The tusks really don't look good and the pus indicates an infection. I want to follow up on that immediately upon arrival in Belgium. And on the subject of that arrival, I would like to get out of here as soon as possible. This week is needed to get the administration in order on site, but that seems more difficult than expected.
Garik and Frosya still have a long journey ahead. They will have to drive around 1,500 miles to Belgium with me and three truck drivers in a truck and a van. To their home. Of those 1,500 miles, half are through Russia and the half through the European Union. During the journey, I am responsible for the walruses. I will feed them regularly with the frozen fish we brought and make sure they are sprayed with water often enough, as we are transporting them dry in boxes. The journey will be comfortable for Garik and Frosya, provided there are no unforeseen circumstances.
But there are.
At the border with Latvia, we're halted.
'Papers no', they say.
'Papers no?' I repeat questioningly.
The Russian in his booth shakes his head complacently.
Bob, one of the truck drivers who is also knowledgeable about Russia

thanks to his Russian wife, chimes in.
'Apparently, the necessary documents are not in order,' he explains. I had already understood that much myself. I get worked up about the slowness and laziness and immediately look at my watch. Garik and Frosya need to be watered and fed again very soon. So I don't want to waste too much time here.
'Ask him what we should do,' I say.
'Go back,' is the answer. My anxiousness is now turning into frustration. Bob parks the truck at a small hotel further down the road.
'I'm sleeping with the animals,' I say as the drivers gather their things to check in at the hotel.
'Are you sure?' asks Geert, one of the other drivers who is in charge of the transport. I nod. I can't leave them alone.
I check on my two walrus friends. I defrost some fish and feed them in their box. They both scarf down about ten fish, It makes me laugh for a moment and forget my misery. Luckily those two treasures don't know what's going on. They are happy with the attention and the fish. I then spray them, and they both drink from the water hose I aim at their mouths. Then we spend the night together. A night that seems to last forever. Every time Garik or Frosya moves, the whole truck shakes and I'm awoken.
The next morning, I drive with Geert straight to the local government's veterinary department, about an hour's drive from the border crossing. Igor is already waiting for us to solve the problem.
'It's Thursday morning now,' he says. 'By this evening, it should be fine.'
But that evening, nothing is fine, just like nothing is fine the following morning. My frustration slowly turns into anger and despair, but I try to hold back. Geert assures me that it won't help to bang the table, quite the contrary. 'But what does help then,
'Geert?' I say firmly. 'We have been standing still in this parking lot for 24 hours with two walruses in the cargo hold of our truck. If this continues any longer, their water and food supply will run out. We need to intervene now, or this will end badly.'
'I'm afraid we have no choice but to wait,' Geert sighs.

But I refuse to believe that.
I review my options and then try something.
'Sorry, Olga', I say a little later on the phone. 'I don't know if you still remember me. I am Tim Bouts, we met at an EAZA meeting.'
'Of course!' she says enthusiastically. That already reassures me. Olga is the director of Moscow Zoo, a zoo that is a member of EAZA, the European Association of Zoos and Aquaria.
'I have a problem,' I explain. 'I'm at the border of Russia and Latvia with two walruses, and we can't leave the country because there seems to be a problem with the paperwork.'
'Send me all the documents and I will see what I can do. But... Tim... If I can give you one piece of advice: drive back to Utrish just to be safe.'
I firmly shake my head.

'We're halfway now, Olga. We've already driven 745 miles. If we turn back now, those walruses may not come out of that truck alive. My visa expires tomorrow. We need to leave the country as soon as possible.'

'I'll do what I can.'
The hours pass agonizingly slow, and I can't do much more than occassionally sit with Garik and Frosya to calm myself.
At 4.30 in the afternoon, I receive a phone call. It's the 'document controller' from Moscow Zoo.
'We have found the issue. A stamp is missing on one of the forms from the local veterinary station in Anapa. Without a stamp, you simply cannot leave the country. You'll have to turn back.'
'No,' I say again, just as firmly.
'Listen. I appreciate your help, but it's not enough. We need to get out of here. And now.'
'I'll see what I can do... The offices close at 5.'

'Then we still have half an hour left,' I say sternly.
At 5.30, I receive another phone call.
'You may proceed, everything is fine.'
'Really?' I can't believe it.
'Yes. We have contacted the veterinarian who forgot to stamp it. He had to fix it right away or he would be fired.'
'Well...' I mutter. But there is no time for pity or understanding. I want to leave.
'We can go!' I shout to Geert and the rest. 'Everything's okay!'
We leave straightaway, and as soon as we get back to the queue at the border crossing we are given priority as animal transport.
'Just keep driving,' I say to Geert, who hesitates due to the many other drivers frustratedly honking their horns as we pass them.
Finally we reach the border crossing, where an official is waiting to speak to us.
'Problem,' he says, after looking at us disapprovingly.
'Goddammit,' I mutter. 'What now?'
Geert wants to ask for more explanation in Russian, but before he can say anything, the official continues in broken English.
'It's a problem of 10,000 euros,' he says.
I don't know whether to laugh or cry. You can't be serious!
'Come on,' I say. 'Isn't it a problem of 5,000 euros?' I suggest.
After some negotiation, it turns out to be just that: a problem of 5,000 euros. An expense I will enter with a somewhat bizarre description in the costs report for this trip.
The border gate opens, and I think I have rarely been as relieved in my life as I am now.
'Drive, Geert. Drive!'
We enter the European Union via Latvia, and the Belgian authorities have already informed the border authorities about our trip. At six in the morning we present all the papers there and Garik and Frosya's microchips are read. Everything is fine. It feels to me as if we are finally home, though we still have 750 miles to drive.
It's already evening when we arrive at Pairi Daiza. A whole team is ready to welcome and guide Garik and Frosya upon their arrival. Yet

I am the only familiar face to them. So I make sure I stay around them, and when they come out of their cage to eat, our adventure is over. The World of Cold just became a little more beautiful and less cold.

25. Just like a real little person

Together with Amandine, one of the regular keepers, I am standing at the large window of the public orangutan enclosure. We want to catch a glimpse of baby Sungai, as he is said to have a problem with his mouth. Because the orangutans do not come backstage on command, we are frontstage for once. Since the arrival of Sungai nine months ago, the orangutan family in Pairi Daiza consists of six animals. The orangutans have all come from different zoos as part of the European breeding program. There are two subspecies, and our subspecies originates from the Indonesian island of Sumatra, but they are a globally endangered species. We have two family groups here in as many enclosures. The birth of Sungai, which is Indonesian for 'river', was therefore very good news for the captive breeding program. Sungai is popular with the public, partly because he is so cute and possibly reminds them of a human baby. The similarities are striking.

'Look! There's the mom with the baby! There! On that bridge!' A grandfather points to where his granddaughter should look, and we turn our heads in the same direction. Sungai is indeed walking over the bridge with mama Sinta. He's hiding his face a little, but I do notice his mouth agape.

'Do you see it?' asks Amandine. That open mouth is actually the reason why the keepers have asked me to come. Sungai is no longer drinking, and that may be the result of a problem with his mouth. I nod. 'It seems like the jaw joint is blocked. I'll contact some specialists to see what we can do,' I reassure Amandine. 'We definitely need to follow up on this urgently.'

We agree that I should be contacted immediately once Sungai appears in the backstage, as it is impossible to enter the orangutan enclosure myself. That would be too dangerous. The next morning I hear Amandine again.

'Sinta is backstage with Sungai!'

I notify the specialists I already spoke to yesterday to come immediately. That includes Bart, a specialized small animal surgeon, and a specialist radiologist, both from the Faculty of Veterinary Medicine. When they arrive, we hurry to the orangutans.

With an injection by hand, Amandine first anesthetizes Sinta. She's is trained for that. She is out quickly. Sungai clings to his sedated mother. I give him a pat on the head and feel the skin on his little arm. He is clearly dehydrated, as his skin is less elastic when I pinch it.

'We need to rehydrate him,' I say. 'And warm him up. I'll try to milk Sinta.'

Sungai is not drinking any more, which means Sinta no longer has milk OR that Sungai simply cannot drink.

'Yes, she has enough milk,' I confirm, while I collect some to feed Sungai, which I manage by simply dripping the milk into his mouth. His jaws remain blocked the whole time, causing his mouth to stay constantly open.

'We're going to sedate him,' I say. That can be done simply with gas anesthesia while he calmly lies on his mom. It's the safest way to put a little one like this under.

Right before I want to put the mask on his face, he looks at me with big, questioning eyes.

'Oh...' says Bart who seems a bit surprised when he sees that. Everyone in the room falls silent, every keeper, every veterinarian.

'Crazy, huh...' Amandine interrupts, used to seeing that look. 'Just like a real little person.'

A shiver runs down my spine. I realize that I'm actually dealing with neonatal care, just like a pediatrician in a hospital. It's very strange to be looked at with such a human gaze by an animal. So strange to see that baby with its mother. They really are just like people. It's not just their body that's similar to that of a human, but also their behaviors, their gaze and their movements.

'He's ready for intubation,' I say when he is out.

'Now the radiologist and surgeon can look at the jaw joint,' I continue, but I am interrupted by the sound of the monitor.

A long, drawn-out beep fills the room. 'Shit.' 'Cardiac arrest,' I say.

I focus and immediately switch to the ABCDEmethod, which is a procedure for providing first aid according to the principle 'treat first what kills first'. In other words: first treat the primary (life-threatening), then the secondary and tertiary (non-direct and non-life-threatening) injuries and disorders. This method not only provides a clear guideline, but also helps to review and possibly treat almost all injuries and disorders.

'A: Airway. Check,' I shout, 'Sungai is intubated.'

'B: Breathing. Ventilation started.'

'C: Circulation. Start chest compressions and call the on-duty first aider to bring the automated external defibrillator (AED).'

I look for a blood vessel to insert a catheter to administer fluid therapy and emergency medication.

Within a few minutes, the AED arrives and we place the electrodes on Sungai. The device analyzes his heart and tells us whether we should continue resuscitation or press the button to administer a shock.

Each time we hear: 'Continue chest compressions.'

We check the pulse oximeter and the blood oxygen saturation remains good, so we continue.

'Come on Sungai...' I think out loud.

I don't want to give up. I can't give up. But when I feel a hand on my shoulder, I realize I have to stop. We have been working for an hour and a half.

'It's no use anymore,' Bart says, resting his hand comfortingly on my shoulder. Only when I look up from Sungai, do I see the sorrow of everyone in the room. Amandine stands with tears in her eyes and her hand in front of her mouth against the wall. Two other keepers are embracing each other.

I look again at Sungai, who lies lifeless on his mother's belly. The image is terrible and leaves no one untouched.

'I'm sorry,' I say, while closing my eyes. I want to apologize, but I also know that this is not my fault. Every sedation carries risks, we know that. We do everything to limit those risks. Something that doesn't always work out...

I am totally dejected, we all are. This is a huge blow and we need to process it. When I leave the room, Amandine gently clings to me. Her eyes are red and watery, her cheeks wet from tears.

'You did what you could,' she says softly. 'Thank you.'

In the midst of her sorrow, the fact that she makes an effort to reassure me means a lot to me.

The next day a press release is sent out to the world.

'In Pairi Daiza, the small Sumatran orangutan Sungai died on Thursday evening. The orangutan was born in the Walloon animal park on October 30, 2018, but suffered from a severe jaw deformity.

Due to additional complications, he could no longer drink from his mother Sinta's breast. As a result, Sungai weakened significantly in a short period of time. He died suddenly. Despite all the veterinarian's efforts to help him regain his strength.

This death is infinitely sad for his parents and for us, even though we know that the early childhood of animals is a period fraught with many dangers. The keepers of our orangutan families are heartbroken. But they will, of course, not give up on Sungai's parents, Sinta and Gempa. Ever since Sungai's passing, they focussed on supporting Sinta during this difficult ordeal no mother should ever have to experience.'

26. She's out

'Tilt a little bit more,' instructs the dentist. 'We need to take a photo of the tusks' roots.' He makes an angle with his hand and Diana, the keeper of walrus Frosya, holds the plate exactly at the same angle against the walrus's head.

'This should work.'

The dentist takes an X-ray of Frosya's teeth then nods when finished. Frosya receives a compliment from the keeper and a fish as reward. As soon as Frosya arrived here, she was trained to have X-rays taken, because her tusks are broken and that can lead to severe infections, even in the brain. A walrus can die from an infection like that, so it is certainly a medical issue that needs to be treated. In Frosya's case, the inflammation is still local, but we have noticed that she occasionally experiences discomfort. When the inflammation flares up, she clearly starts having more difficulty eating, so we definitely shouldn't wait any longer.

At the first meeting with Frosya in Russia, the keepers and veterinarian were already rinsing the tusks, and that was also the first thing they taught me as part of the daily routine. Since her arrival in Belgium, the keepers have been doing that twice a day. I check the openings weekly by putting my finger in and smelling them: sometimes the inflammation is quite clean and I don't smell anything, while other times it's terribly pus-filled with an equally terrible smell. To accurately determine the condition of those teeth and the inflammation, an X-ray is urgently needed. It shows that the inflammation around the teeth is advanced. We see a clear inflammatory reaction around the root with damage to the bone around it. The tusks need to be removed, there is no other option.

For us, that's where the search begins, because there aren't many people experienced in operating on walrus teeth. I know one, a human dentist in London, but they have an extremely long waiting time and can only come in six months at the earliest. The dentist who took the

X-rays recommends a dentist who is also a veterinarian: Cedric, a South African who has operated on walruses worldwide and extracted teeth. The fact that he is a veterinarian and not a human dentist, I find to be an extra bonus.

'I'm coming,' he says immediately when we present him with Frosya's case.

I will take care of the anesthesia myself, but not alone. For a walrus, this is an extremely complicated procedure. Marine mammals like a walrus have a diving reflex. The diving reflex or underwater reflex is an innate reflex that causes the breathing to automatically stop when an animal's face or head goes underwater. At the same time, the blood pressure drops so that only vital organs are supplied with blood and the heart rate slows down. Some anesthesia products trigger that reflex, but if the diving reflex were to occur during anesthesia, the animal would stop breathing and could die.

I don't want to take any risks, so for extra reinforcement, I'm calling in Alex, a colleague anesthesiologist from Latvia specialized in wildlife anesthesia, and Charlotte, a friend anesthesiologist from the University of Ghent, because they have an anesthesia machine that can also be used for ventilation.

'We split up as agreed,' I say before we start the operation with the whole team. There have been several meetings and we have agreed that Alex and Charlotte will be by the walrus's head to monitor the anesthesia, while I will be by the tail flipper to insert catheters into the superficial blood vessels. This way, we can administer fluids and have a life-saving access to the blood to potentially administer additional anesthesia products or other medication when needed.

I shoot a dart in Frosya's rear end with midazolam and butorphanol to calm her down, but it doesn't work well enough.

'I'll try again,' I say as I administer a second shot. 'We're seeing the first effects of the sedation, now we can administer ketamine to induce her.'

'She's out,' I say after about ten minutes.

'Now we can intubate.' I use a tracheal tube for intubation. I open the mouth and attach a cord to the lower and upper jaw. One keeper stands over Frosya and pulls the upper jaw up while another keeper pulls the lower jaw down. Now I can reach into Frosya's mouth with my hand to intubate her windpipe. I feel her sharp teeth digging into the skin of my hand and arm, but try to ignore this. My arm is all the way in Frosya's mouth almost up to my elbow, and suddenly I feel the fleshy larynx, the opening of the windpipe. I insert my index and middle fingers into this opening and open the larynx. With my other hand, I slide the tube along my arm between the two fingers in the opening. This better be done in one smooth motion, as there is always the risk of the diving reflex occurring.

'Done it!' I say relieved. But this is only step one. 'Start the ventilation.'

From then on, it's a nervous wait.

'The anesthesia machine is connected, ventilation started,' I hear. 'Pulse oximeter on the tongue, capnograph ready; heart rate stable, CO_2 stable.'

I nod to my colleagues and try to breathe a sigh of relief. I notice that I hold my breath until I feel like everything is under control.

It's really exciting to do something like this, precisely because it's so exceptional. Though, that's also the reason why it causes so much stress.

While my two colleagues take over at the front, I go to the back. I spray the flipper with warm water so that the veins expand and I can insert a catheter to start the fluid therapy.

'So, lift her up then, huh?' Alex indicates the next step of our procedure. The tusks are rooted in the upper jaw. The dentist would have easy access to that upper jaw by laying the patient on its back, but that's not an option with Frosya. By lying on her back, too much weight would be put on the lungs, which would make breathing difficult. We leave Frosya lying there as she is, on her stomach, but

we lift her up until she is somewhat elevated. This way, the dentist can work better.
Though it's easier said than done, lifting a walrus weighing over 1,300 pounds. With some ingenuity and the help of a few pallets, we manage to get Frosya half a meter off the ground.
'That should do the trick,' the dentist confirms. He immediately starts working with his equipment specially developed for these procedures, so he can remove the tusks in the best and fastest way possible.
'The good news is that it's all so rotten that it comes off easily,' he says while working.
'The bad news, at least for me, is that this might stink.' And he is right. There is a strong rotten smell coming from Frosya's mouth, indicating the extent to which the infection is festering. In just under three quarters of an hour, the tusks are out completely. The dentist quickly rinses the area and administers antibiotics.
'I think we're done,' he concludes.
His work may be done, but I still have to wake Frosya from the anesthesia with the rest of the team.
With just as much effort and invention, we manage to lower her again.
'Breathing is fine,' I hear again.
'Heart rate stable.'
'CO_2 stable.'
I administer a drug to help her wake up again. We leave the tube in the trachea a little longer, until we're certain she can breathe and swallow on her own. If we remove it too fast, we lose all control if the diving reflex still occurs. Only when she seems alert again and responds well to us and her surroundings, a burden is lifted off my shoulders. And that goes for everyone within the team, even for the keepers who could only watch during the procedure. Keepers of marine mammals are highly specialized in what they do; they know their animals exceptionally well, precisely because they realize how rare their animals are. Because anesthesia is never the first option for an examination, they train frequently on taking blood samples and

other procedures that preferably happen without anesthesia. When the animal does have to be put under, keepers usually have little or no experience with it. They need to let go of control at that moment, and we need to take over.

27. Fashionable disease

Ninety percent of the day I am on my knees on the ground. That's often the best way to study animals, exactly what I am doing with Dana at the zoo. Dana is one of our lionesses who has been living in the park for years. She arrived with Danny, her mate. Both have been real crowd favorites from the start. Dana has been experiencing various symptoms for several days, which Puria, one of her regular keepers, is now listing for me.
'She stopped eating, breathes heavily, and just sits in a corner of her enclosure.'
Indeed, she does seem lethargic to me: sleepy, lacking energy and indifferent to any activity. It's definitely not how a lion is supposed to behave.
'What can you do?' Puria asks a bit impatiently. I don't blame him for that impatience. He wants to cure his lion and can only count on me for that.
'I could prescribe an antibiotic. But since she's not eating, she will also not take oral antibiotics.'
Puria nods worriedly. 'Can it be administered with a syringe?'
'No. Dana weighs 330 pounds. The largest darts we can shoot only have a capacity of 0.34ounces. That also limits us, as that amount is only sufficient for an animal weighing up to 220 pounds.
I consider my options.
'I will have to treat her under anesthesia, which is the best and only option in this case.'

The lions know me very well as 'the man with the gun' by now. So from the moment I arrive, they would rather eat me alive.

When I dart them, they look me in the eyes, roaring, and attack towards the fence. The adrenaline rushes through my body and it's difficult to keep my gun steady, every time.

After I have sedated her from a distance with my dart gun, and she tears apart the dart in her jaws, I can conduct a full examination thanks to our mobile equipment.

I start by inserting a thermometer into her rectum to measure her temperature. Dana clearly has a high fever, which also partly explains her rapid and shallow breathing. I hear a sandpaper-like sound with the stethoscope at the level of the lungs and the nose is also blocked. That's a problem for any feline, because once their sense of smell is obstructed, they stop eating.

I start my differential diagnosis, so I can differentiate between different diseases. To do this, I actually create a list of possible diagnoses that fit the animal's symptoms in order of likelihood. Then I can systematically work through that list by a series of tests. First, I want to rule out a viral infection, because two types of flu called para-influenza and Calicivirus have already been diagnosed in wild felines. COVID has also been detected in tigers at the American Bronx Zoo.

I choose a suitable spot to draw blood on the inside of Dana's hind leg, as the most superficial blood vessels are located there. When I insert the catheter, blood immediately flows across my hand and I connect the syringe to draw about 0.70 ounces of blood. I collect enough blood to test the serum for antibodies and perform a general blood check. After that, I connect an IV before continuing with my tests.

Then I take a tester to do a nasal swab. I insert it deep and long enough into both nostrils to perform a PCR analysis for Covid. Throughout the entire Covid period, I have had a tester in my nose many times, so I know how terribly annoying it is. Luckily, Dana is under anesthesia and doesn't feel anything.

'I'm going to try and patch you up, girl,' I say, even though she doesn't hear me and wouldn't even understand me. But I want to reassure her and myself. Because I'm still not sure what's going on, I administer another fever-reducing medicine directly into the blood

and a long-acting antibiotic under her skin.
I pat her on the side encouragingly once, to make it clear that she did well, and then stand up. My legs feel stiff. I rub my hand over my thighs as I look at Dana. I feel sorry for her. So impressive and yet so weak.
A few days later, Dana still isn't eating and she is still lethargic. The results of the investigations are in. I will also inform Puria right away.
'Good news and bad news,' I say.
'Do I want to know?' He shakes his head.
'Dana tested negative for all common respiratory viruses known in felines. That's the good news. But... she has tested positive for Covid.'
'That's the bad news...' Puria continues.
It's just a few weeks after the national lockdown and Covid is a 'fashionable' disease everywhere at the moment, so I remain sceptical. However, she does test strongly positive and her symptoms match the typical Covid pathology.
'How on earth did she get infected?' Puria wonders.
Now I have to shake my head.
'We probably won't get an answer to that. Either a visitor or keeper has transmitted the virus to Dana, or perhaps the disease is present in other animals. Either way, she must remain isolated from the other lions.' Lions are group animals, so Dana's not happy about her being separated, but we can't afford other lions getting infected by her. So it remains a necessary evil.
'And now?' Puria wants as many answers as possible, as quickly as possible. But I can hardly give them at the moment. There is currently no specific treatment for Covid, neither for humans nor for animals.
'She definitely needs to continue treatment because she still isn't eating.'
'Another anesthesia then?'
I nod.
Once again, I give Dana a boost with extra fluid and antibiotics. After that, we have to wait once more.
A few days later, Puria calls me. 'She's eating again!'

It seems that the acute infection is under control, although she continues to test positive for Covid.

Dana is closely monitored, but after about ten days, I'm armed with my gun to sedate her for the third time. Dana is deteriorating again. I go through the same routine this time: blood draw, nasal swab, and administering fluids and antibiotics. The results of the swab indicate that Dana still tests positive for Covid, but not as strongly as before. The fever has also gone and the breathing has normalized. So something else is going on, and the blood sample proves it: the lion is suffering from acute kidney failure. This confuses me. Is this related to the Covid infection? I want and need to be able to rule that out, and to do that I immerse myself in the existing literature and turn to human doctors. They have been dealing with the virus for a while now and know more about it than I do.

And what do you know? Most Covid deaths occur after kidney failure. So it is not the acute respiratory phase that leads to death, it is the second sub-acute phase with kidney problems that is fatal. This knowledge is extremely valuable for human doctors but also for me in the case of Dana.

I need to get those kidneys working again, and in humans, this is done with prolonged fluid therapy, but I can't keep Dana under anesthesia for hours, let alone days.

'I'll have to go on my knees again,' I say to Puria, who knows that I mean Dana will have to be put under anesthesia again.

I try to administer as much fluid as possible intravenously and subcutaneously, flushing her kidneys and removing the toxins.

And it helps. After seeing or speaking to Puria each day, it's a phone call on the seventh day that confirms it: 'Dana seems fully recovered, she is eating with gusto again and shows interest when I call her name as I enter,' he says. Puria and I have had a lot of contact lately, but it's the first time I really hear relief in his voice. Something that relieves me too.

Because of this case, I realize how important it is that we have identified those two phases, the respiratory phase and the renal failure phase. Because we have been closely monitoring Dana from the start, the data we have collected is of great value. This is a breakthrough, not only for Dana, but also for researchers and veterinarians.

28. New mother

We're all watching the monitor showing walrus Tania. Tania is from the Oceanogràfic Aquarium of the City of Arts and Sciences in Valencia, Spain. She temporarily moved to Tierpark und Tropen Aquarium Hagenbeck in the German city of Hamburg to mate with Odin, the only male walrus in Europe capable of reproducing. When she was found to be pregnant, she was transferred to the walrus enclosure at Pairi Daiza. And now she is in labor.

'She slept from midnight to three o'clock, then she was restless for an hour, before sleeping again until the shift change,' Dana, the walruses' chief keeper, informs me.

'That's right, after the switch she slept until an hour ago. Since then, she has been working pretty hard. I don't think we'll have to wait much longer for the birth,' a colleague keeper chimes in.

On the monitor, we can see how restless Tania is becoming. We see contractions of her body, which must be labor pains. They might be right: that little one is going to be born soon.

This will be the highlight of an intense period during which I have been monitoring Tania. A walrus pregnancy is very rare and not much is known about it. Walruses, like giant pandas, have delayed implantation, which means that mating and fertilization of the eggs occur at a certain point, with the embryo being implanted only later. It can take up to four months, months during which the walrus is not officially pregnant. The total pregnancy lasts 15 to 16 months, but you could also say one year if you discount the unofficial pregnancy phase. From an aquarium in Canada where two walruses were pregnant, I received a publication with not a whole of information: the age of the fetus and the expected birth date can be determined from the circumference of the rib cage on a walrus ultrasound. During the last months, I also drew blood to perform a progesterone test: the more the progesterone level dropped, the more the end of pregnancy was in sight.

'Her water has broken!' someone suddenly shouts. We all immediately dive towards the monitor. And indeed: there is a puddle of water around Tania. She has been kept separate on a dry dock for several days, because a baby walrus cannot swim immediately after birth. So it's important to let that young be born in dry surroundings.
Now it's just a matter of minutes. We stare at the monitor and switch cameras every time Tania turns, to make sure we don't miss anything.
'There!' Jose calls out. 'I already see the back flipper!'
Little by little, the body slides out until we see the head.
'She did it..' I say as we embrace each other. 'She did it!'
'Welcome, little Floki!' Emotions are running high, because we have been looking forward to this moment for a long time.
'She did a perfect job,' I conclude. Now we can go to the dry dock to see the little one. While we are watching that beautiful new life, Tania is trying to activate her young. She pushes it away with a hard blow, sending it hurtling across the ground.
'Oh!' one of the keepers calls out in surprise, but this kind of activation is normal. A walrus can take a hit.
'Now Floki still needs to drink. Come on...' I whisper to myself.
But that doesn't happen straightaway. Tania keeps crawling around nervously and Floki doesn't get the chance to latch onto the nipples. One of the keepers is starting to worry.
'Should we help?'
I shake my head. 'We'll give them some more time.'
But time appears to be insufficient. The baby refuses to drink. Because of our limited knowledge, we don't know the implications of hand-rearing a walrus calf. I decide to call Teresa, the veterinarian from Valencia. They also have limited knowledge of baby walruses, but a vast amount of knowledge about walruses in general. Maybe together we'll get somewhere.
'Try giving Valium,' Teresa says.
'It's possible that Tania, as a new mother, doesn't know what to do and therefore keeps turning around to look for the young one instead of calmly lying down and offering her nipples. Valium will alleviate that 'restlessness' in her, allowing her to let her young drink.'

'We will feed her and administer a low dose of Valium,' I tell the team.
Tania gratefully devours her piece of fish and not long after she visibly becomes more relaxed. Instead of nervously crawling around, she lets herself sink onto her side, making her nipples more accessible to Floki.
'Yes...' I say. 'Come on, little one.'
The calf crawls towards Tania and immediately starts drinking. Greedily even, the milk running down the corners of its mouth.
'Yes,' I say again. 'She did it.'
Tania and Floki are doing well, and a year later we send Petrushka to Germany for a new attempt at fertilization. Petrushka returns from that trip pregnant. For the second time, we can monitor such an exceptional walrus pregnancy and have the opportunity to expand our knowledge.
Everything is going well and we are not worrying too much during all those months, there's no need to. Until the moment the keepers call me late in the evening to tell me that Petrushka is in labor.
I get into my car and hurry to the enclosure to be on standby, in case something goes wrong. When I arrive, Petrushka is writhing restlessly on the ground, behaving as if she could give birth at any moment.
'She's already pushing,' one of the keepers remarks. Petrushka does indeed push and immediately something comes out of her vagina.
'The baby is here!' someone shouts confidently.
'That's not a calf,' I say, worried.
'What?'
'No. That's not a calf. That's vaginal mucosa being pushed outwards, indicating that the calf is likely positioned incorrectly. I'm calling my colleagues in Germany.'
I quickly explain what is happening and receive the reassurance that a team will depart immediately. But we can't wait for that.
'Can't you administer oxytocin' the keeper asks. Oxytocin induces uterine contractions, but should only be used when the birth canal is clear. If this is not the case, the uterus can rupture. The vaginal mucosa protruding outward makes me suspect that oxytocin is contraindicated here.

'But Petrushka is straining and in pain, that can't be good. Do something!' The concern is rising and I need to intervene. But how? Suddenly Petrushka turns around with her back to the bars, just close enough for me to reach the birth canal with my arm. I lie on the ground so I can feel inside her vagina with my hand. Up to my shoulder, as far as I can reach, I try to feel the baby, but I feel nothing. I don't feel any baby, not even at my fingertips.
Shaking my head, I look at the team, standing helplessly at a distance. 'I can't reach the baby. The only solution now is to wait until the specialists from Germany arrive and then see if we can perform a cesarean section,' I say with a trembling voice.
By morning, Petrushka becomes very restless. I realize things are definitely going wrong now. I continue to observe her from a distance and notice that she suddenly starts having convulsions. Her body shakes back and forth while she moans. One last spasm and then she lies motionless. She is dead.
'My tools!' I call out without hesitation. I don't let emotions overwhelm me, and want to act immediately. I need to perform an emergency C-section, otherwise we will lose not only Petrushka but also her calf.
Diana rushes towards me with the necessary tools and I cut open Petruschka's belly. I remove the fetus from the womb and immediately feel that there is no life in it.
'God damn it...' I curse. In the blink of an eye, we lost a mother and her calf.
When the German team arrives, it is no longer to assist with a birth, but to perform an autopsy. By doing this, we can understand what happened: the baby was lying with its back towards the birth canal, which is called a transverse position, stopping any movement when Petruschka pushed. She tried so hard that she pushed out not the baby, but the mucosa, the lining of the vagina. The fetus died before it could be born, and Petrushka contracted blood poisoning from the deceased fetus in the womb, which proved fatal to her.
When I rejoin the keepers, everyone is disconsolate. It's terrible to have to lose an animal, especially in such circumstances. Especially

when you are standing by and watching, without being able to do anything to help. Now the emotions are welling up for me too. I'm devastated. The same team with which we celebrated the birth of Floki last year is now in deep mourning.

Petrushka and the young one were donated to the anatomy department of the Faculty of Veterinary Medicine at Ghent University, and as a team we are trying to come to terms with this loss. We have to. We're definitely allowed to be human, but we must also remain professional, for the sake of the other animals. Life in the World of the Cold continues.

One year later, I receive a message from Jonah. He's at the anatomical museum of the Faculty of Veterinary Medicine and has seen something special there.

'Petrushka and her calf are displayed here. They have been given a second life,' I read on the screen. Then two photos arrive: the skeletons of Petrushka and her young hang centrally from the ceiling of the museum. I gulp. The fact that mother and calf can still serve science in this way pleases me. If we can save other walruses through the experience of their death, that's even better.

The human zoo

Insects, spiders, reptiles, birds, mammals... In a zoo, there are so many different animals to be found, and each animal group is in turn subdivided into hundreds of species. This makes working as a veterinarian in a zoo incredibly interesting, every day. A group of animals that everyone typically finds fascinating is undoubtedly the monkeys. Scientifically, they are called the non-human primates. If there are non-human primates, there must also be human primates. And that's us, humans.

The human being is a very interesting species in itself, but in my opinion also the most difficult to deal with. Just like they say that owners often resemble their dogs, I can make that comparison in a zoo as well. Because many people seem to resemble the animals there as well. There are even hierarchies like those found in social animals that live in groups. After all those years of working in various zoos in different countries and cultures, I can conclude that certain positions often require specific personality traits.

As far as I'm concerned, a zoo is therefore twofold, with on the one hand an animal zoo and on the other hand the human zoo.

The CEO is often a polar bear. The polar bear is a charismatic animal that is seen as an emblem of nature conservation, a symbol of climate change. Most people love the polar bear and admire it. But it's also a top predator that isn't afraid to attack, a loner that roams an ice-cold territory alone.

The zoological director is often a silverback. This is the

gorilla that leads a group of gorillas. He is the undisputed leader in his group and ensures that everyone carries out their task in the group. He corrects where necessary, but is gentle when the group is functioning properly. But woe betide any outsider that attacks the group. He then becomes aggressive and will protect his group with his life.

The keepers are worker ants, always busy working for the colony. Without a keeper, there is no zoo. They are the backbone of the zoo, but unfortunately are all too often invisible. Just like those ants. In every zoo where I have worked, I have met incredibly passionate keepers. People who do everything for their animals every day, rain, snow, or shine.

Rhinos are people who just storm through everything, without taking into account the collateral damage this could cause. They are often hard workers but poor communicators. And in their hard work, often more harm than good is done.

The truly bad guys are the hyenas, which we know from the movie *The Lion King*. These are overambitious and often young people who want to climb up at the expense of others. They can hang around someone and bite that person regularly to weaken them. And when that happens, they attack. The vultures also join in at that moment to get a piece of the action, literally and figuratively. Unfortunately, you'll encounter these people often and, even though you know what's coming, you still get bitten now and again.

Then there are the snakes who slither around management just to be seen, the sloths who would rather be lazy than tired, and the bullfrogs who need no further explanation.

But it's not all bad. In all those years, I have also seen people with good animal qualities, people with the wisdom of the elephant, the pride and strength of the eagle, and the playfulness of the otters.

As a veterinarian, I have more affinity with animals than with people anyway. That means I have had to learn a lot, often through trial and error. I have run a zoo for a long time, which means that I had to run both the human and the animal zoo. My experience has taught me that the first is often more difficult than the second.

29. Declared dead

Two keepers are holding back a tortoise with all their might while she's trying to escape the stool we put her on.
'She can't get away now,' someone says, as the animal thrashes with its legs as if it could escape at any moment.
Isabella, the 220-pound Aldabra tortoise we are dealing with, is one of the largest land tortoises in our zoo and certainly one of our oldest animals, estimated to be sixty years old. The natural habitat of the Aldabra tortoise is limited to the Aldabra Atoll of the Seychelles and some islands beyond, which explains why they are also known as the Seychelles giant tortoise. In the wild, there are several thousands of these tortoises.
Isabella is leading a very good life in her fully adapted enclosure at the zoo, but she had stopped eating a few days ago, which could indicate a serious underlying issue. Since reptiles are cold-blooded, symptoms of disease are not noticed until late. When we detect something abnormal, it is therefore best to intervene quickly. In an earlier phase, it was decided to administer antibiotics, but so far it hasn't changed the situation. A blood sample is now needed to make a diagnosis and find an appropriate treatment. However, it's not easy taking blood from a tortoise. This specimen is extremely large and strong, so it's not possible to just hold it. She would just wriggle free. Hence the stool that at best makes her flounder with discomfort, but otherwise keeps her in place. There are some veins in the neck that could be pricked, but so far I have not been able to get a tortoise like Isabella to stick out her neck on command. On the contrary. The only possible place for a successful blood draw is therefore in the vein in its tail. To prick that vein, I need to keep the tail straight and insert the needle at an angle of 30 to 45 degrees in the middle of the tail, after which suction is applied to the syringe when withdrawing the needle until blood flows into the syringe.
'Any success?' Pascal, one of the keepers, asks.

'No, not yet,' I say. 'Give me another minute.'
Isabella is a stubborn little creature, but I can also be persistent. And persistence pays off.
'Done it,' I say relieved. After several attempts, a usable blood sample is successfully taken.
'She can go back to ground level,' I say. 'Ready?'
'Ready,' they all say in unison.
'One, two, three...'
With the three of us, we carefully lift the tortoise from the stool to put her on the ground and let her crawl away.
'That one needs a minute to recover,' Pascal remarks, while Isabella remains motionless for a moment.
'Just like us,' I joke.
I wait for the results of the blood sample, which indicate a clearly elevated calcium level. Reptiles with an elevated calcium level often have a problem with egg laying. In reptiles, it's important to distinguish between egg stasis and oocyst stasis. Oocyst stasis must always be resolved surgically, while egg stasis can often be treated with medication. To know what we are dealing with here, a correct diagnosis is needed first and foremost. Normally, an X-ray examination can provide clarity, but that huge shield doesn't let any X-ray radiation through. An ultrasound then.
'One, two, three...' I say again, this time to lift Isabella back onto the stool to take that ultrasound. There is only one accessible spot for that, and that is in front of the hind leg, in a cavity between the upper and lower shell. It takes some more juggling, as we need to pull the hind leg backwards; and of course Isabella resists, requiring two people to hold the leg in place. But the ultrasound does provide clarity: the image shows dozens of oocysts, indicating that Isabella is suffering from oocyst stasis, where the eggs or, in this case, oocysts are still in the ovaries and not in the uterus.
The only way to solve this is sterilization. Now, I have sterilized tortoises before, but never such a huge Aldabra tortoise. Normally, I open the ventral shield using a plaster saw to perform the sterilization and then glue the shield back in place. But for that, the shield

must not be too thick, which of course turns out to be the case after taking some measurements. So I will have to come up with something else.

Surfing the Internet for more references or possibilities, I open my Facebook page just for distraction. While I aimlessly scroll through all the posts, my gaze lingers on a post by Bart, a friendly professor from Ghent University. In his post, he talks about a case where he performs an endoscopic procedure on a dog. During that procedure, a veterinarian only uses instruments and a camera that are inserted into the body through one or more small incisions. This is also known as minimally invasive surgery. Next to the operating table is a magnified screen displaying the camera image. It's actually keyhole surgery, quite an improvement from a non-endoscopic spay, which requires opening up the animal's abdomen several inches.

'That's it,' I think out loud. I call him right away.

'Bart, do you feel like extracting oocysts from a tortoise under endoscopic guidance?' I ask, after a brief introduction.

The response follows just as quickly. 'Well...I've never done that, but yes, I would like to, for sure. Let me read up on tortoise endoscopy so I'm up to date with the latest techniques.'

A few days later Pascal and I drive to the Faculty of Veterinary Medicine in Merelbeke, with Isabella in the trunk, in high spirits. Bart will perform the sterilization, and I will take care of the anesthesia. My specialty, so not necessarily an easy task.

'One, two, three…' Once again, Isabella has to be placed on a stool against her will, and this time she's not cooperating much at all.

'You'd think third time lucky,' Pascal winks. But alas.

Once in position, Isabella is again difficult to prick, but eventually I manage to find a blood vessel and inject propofol, an intravenous anesthetic for administering general anesthesia.

'Guys, it took a while. But she's out,' I conclude after a few minutes.

'Ready for intubation,' I nod. We open the mouth by pulling both jaws open and I insert a tube into her windpipe.

The intubation is necessary because we will be putting pressure on the lungs shortly. Isabella needs to lie on her back, causing all the abdominal organs in the cavity under the shell to press on the lungs.

'Shall I count this time,' Pascal asks, while he's preparing to flip Isabella on her back with us.

'Go ahead,' I say.

Once she's lying on her back in front of us, everything is ready for the procedure. Bart will make an incision in front of the hind leg to reach the ovaries.

'I will start by opening the abdominal cavity,' Bart announces. He makes an incision and then inserts the camera. As soon as he does that, we're startled by a 'Beeeeeeep.'

We hear and see the breathing flatlining. Isabella is not doing anything anymore. I immediately search for a heartbeat, first with the doppler and then with an ultrasound, but I find nothing. I keep trying, but it seems futile.

'Nothing?' Bart asks hurriedly.

'Nothing.' I shake my head.

'Then we've lost her...' Bart concludes. Frustrated, he drops his hands.

'No,' I reply. 'No,' I repeat, to make it clear for myself as well. 'We're dealing with a reptile here, don't forget. Bart, you continue the procedure. Is that okay? Then I'll continue with the ventilation.'

Meanwhile, the monitors show nothing. The only thing left is that beeping. Technically speaking, Isabella is dead.

Bart looks at me questioningly for a moment, sees that I am determined to continue, and then springs back into action.

'Good...' he says.

Pascal looks a bit helpless. He doesn't dare to do anything, say anything.

'Reptiles have been known to sometimes 'freeze',' I explain. 'When they do that, sometimes they only have a heartbeat once per hour and you often can no longer detect their breathing. I would like to assume that Isabella is currently freezing.'

Pascal nods, he seems hopeful. Just like me.

With eyes and mouth wide open, I watch as Bart does what he needs to do through a large sleeve; it's fantastic to see.

'Look here,' he says. 'Oophoritis.' On the image, I now see a massive amount of oocysts, too many to count, with abscesses on them. So high time to remove these cysts. He removes the right ovary and we put the cysts in a bowl that we weigh: Over 3 pounds of infected cysts. Now we go to the left, where we get the same view. Once again, the cysts are removed and then weighed. 2.6 pounds. Man oh man, this was really necessary or our tortoise definitely would have died from infection. Although there's also the chance she might not survive this either.

'Is she breathing again?' Bart asks as he finishes the procedure.

'Not yet,' I say, without drawing any conclusions from that.

'That animal is dead, Tim,' Bart repeats. But I keep shaking my head.

'She's coming back to the zoo with me,' I decide. With a nod, I indicate to Pascal that we are going to transport her again.

It's quite a hassle and we have to count to three a few times again, but a little later we are on our way back to the zoo.

'You drive,' I say to Pascal. 'I'll continue with the ventilation.' Pascal has long realized that he shouldn't ask me any further questions, but should just trust me. Also when I ask him to drive the car so I can ventilate a tortoise. Isabella is still intubated and not awake, so I can occasionally blow air into the endotracheal tube to help her breathe. However, Pascal also starts to doubt a little as we arrive at the zoo with Isabella, who still shows no sign of life.

'She seems pretty dead...' he offers cautiously before I decide what to do now.

'We'll drop her off at the clinic and see what she does in the morning.' To which, I catch: 'If she does something...' He seems to be losing hope, and to be honest, I'm starting to have doubts too, but I won't tell him that.

In the morning, I arrive at the clinic first. I open the door curiously, but I immediately see that Isabella is still lying in the same place where we left her yesterday.

'Okay. She's dead then,' I mutter disappointedly. I had such high

hopes. It was really possible. Isabella could have gone into freeze mode just to endure everything and then bounce back. But unfortunately... I was wrong.
I'm really not looking forward to making that phone call. Not because I was wrong; I can handle that just fine. But now I have to tell a keeper that his animal has passed away.
'Pascal,' I say. 'She's dead. You can come and get her. I'm sorry.'
'I'll come after lunch,' he confirms. 'Oh well... we knew anyway,' he tries, without making me feel guilty. And perhaps I can't be blamed for preferring to believe in a happy ending.
Around ONE in the afternoon, my phone rings. It's Pascal.
'Tim?' He sounds confused. 'I am at the clinic. Isabella is walking around here, you know that, right? Or not?'
'What?!'
I let out a laugh of disbelief and hurry to the clinic. Pascal is waiting for me with a big grin and his eyes widen when he opens the door of the clinic for me.
'Incredible,' I whisper. 'Incredible!' Isabella has indeed moved and is now sitting a few feet further than this morning. She was declared dead, but is now alive and kicking!
'You can take her away for real now,' I say excitedly. 'But keep her away from the public a little longer. She must now be fed well and recover.'
A few days later, it turns out that Isabella still isn't eating well, but we solve this by giving her a medicine orally that stimulates her appetite. Isabella can be considered a miracle tortoise, an animal that has risen from the dead. Even more so, she is proof that the recovery of reptiles occurs differently than believed, without breathing, without a heartbeat. But still with a good outcome.

30. We have bad news

I insert my hand into Mala the elephant's rectum and slide it further past my elbow to remove as much dung from the intestine as possible. But soon I notice that there is no dung to remove.

'You see,' says Rob, Mala's keeper. He looks a bit lost, garden hose in hand. 'She has deteriorated very rapidly in a short period of time, she no longer produces any muck.' She also hasn't eaten or drunk anymore.'

I nod.

It's clear Mala has an acute problem. Mala is 55 years old and a real crowd favorite. She transferred from the Hamburg zoo and quickly developed into the absolute matriarch of the group. She loves the attention from her keepers and the public. But now she is severely dehydrated and constipated. The first thing that needs to happen in cases of dehydration is hydration. The treatment involves administering as much fluid as possible. Usually this can be done effectively with an IV, but an adult elephant can't possibly receive enough fluid through the blood vessels alone. On the contrary. Once a day, Mala will need to be fully sedated, after which she will receive an IV and all other necessary medication; and she will also need to be rehydrated at least three times a day, without sedation, by administering fluid rectally with a garden hose, so that we can give several hundred liters at once.

After giving the injection with a cocktail of two medications and successfully sedating Mala, I insert several catheters into the blood vessels of the ears and hind legs, so that we can set up different infusions together to get as much fluid as possible into the blood as quickly as possible. First, a hypertonic saline solution has to be administered. This solution contains a very high concentration of salt, causing extra fluid to be drawn into the bloodstream to dilute this salt. By giving relatively little fluid, a lot of fluid is thereby drawn into the bloodstream, causing Mala to rehydrate faster.

After that, she receives a fluid through an IV with a composition similar to that of her own blood. She also receives additional fluid therapy through the rectum, as elephants can absorb fluids well in that area thanks to large blood vessels.

I gesture to Rob to hand me the garden hose he's been holding the whole time.

'Turn on the faucet,' I say. I feel the water moving through the garden hose, and eventually fluid flows into Mala's rear. Normally, it's enough to insert the garden hose and then remove it again after a few minutes. After that, the water would simply flow out again. But nothing happens with Mala.

'It's been three to four minutes now,' Rob remarks. 'Not a drop comes back out. Is that normal?'

'I'll keep going for a little while longer,' I say, but it doesn't seem to alleviate his concerns.

When I stop, a few minutes later, Rob takes a step closer.

'It's not good, right?' He sounds worried, but I can't reassure him because I'm also worried, very worried.

'No, Rob, this is not good at all. No water is flowing back, I've never seen this before. Either she's extremely dehydrated, or – and that would be terrible news – her intestine has burst and all that water is leaking into her abdominal cavity. If that's the case, then I fear for her life. We'll have to repeat this procedure a few more times,' I explain. 'Then we can evaluate which of the two options is most likely.'

After finishing the fluid therapy, I will give Mala some additional medication. She gets metoclopramide injected into her bloodstream to get her bowels moving again and painkillers for the abdominal pain caused by constipation, which we also call colic, as in horses. We also decide to administer lactulose, a human medication used for constipation. We give up to 3 ounces in her mouth three times a day.

I also examine her teeth. An elephant has seven sets of molars over its lifetime. With those molars, it sometimes grinds up to over 400 pounds of grass, branches, leaves and bark per day. The molars wear down and shift forward slowly as new ones come in behind them. But after seven sets it's over, and the animal has to gradually adapt its diet to its teeth. If that doesn't happen, the elephant will stop eating and deteriorate rapidly. We have known for some time that Mala is also on her last set of teeth and that at some point she would have difficulties, but no one could predict exactly when we should adjust her diet to prevent problems. Her teeth show clear flattening and some cracks, so it's clear that the initial problem lies here. If Mala survives, we will have to adjust her diet to this new reality.

After repeating the entire procedure a few times – three days during which I reach into the elephant up to three times a day and do a colonic irrigation – nothing changes. Mala still doesn't eat or drink, and she also does not produce any dung.

She is going to die. That's what everyone fears, including Rob and me.

'I fear the worst,' Rob says as we prepare everything for yet another flush. 'We need to keep the public informed. Otherwise there will be a massive shock.' He hangs his head. He is heartbroken. The true Mala fans are worried because she hasn't been seen in public for several days.

'And yet we keep going,' I argue. I don't want to give up that easily. This stops only when Mala herself decides to stop.

'I'll have our press office post a message on our Facebook page,' Rob says softly.

When I get home that evening, I open my Facebook account. I immediately see Mala's announcement appear on the screen.

'We have bad news. Our elephant matriarch, Mala, is not doing well. Mala is 55 years old and shows severe symptoms of colic. Our veterinarian and the elephant team are watching over her day and night, doing everything they can to make her better, but it doesn't look good. Old elephants cannot digest their food properly anymore due to their teeth deteriorating, which is likely the case here. Hopefully we can share a positive update soon. We will keep you informed, but we do ask our visitors to remain calm around the elephants as the whole team is busy trying to save Mala.'

Under the post, hundreds of people have left a comment.

'Poor Mala.' 'Hopefully she makes it.' 'Do your best.' 'Come on, Mala!'

Among all those reactions, there are a few that stand out to me. A spiritual healer explains that Mala's energy is out of balance and that she can restore everything to equilibrium. An acupuncturist also offers his services. A whole bunch of people want to come and help save Mala. But I don't have the energy to sift through all those responses to distinguish between well-meaning quackery and genuine help. I trust that we have enough expertise in-house to help Mala recover. And I hope I will never regret not calling on those others.

The next morning I receive a phone call on my way to the zoo. 'Rob – elephants' is displayed on the screen.

It can't be... I gulp and hesitate for a moment before answering. It's already the fourth day that Mala has not been eating or drinking. Did he call to say she passed away?

Before I can greet him, he speaks.

'She's drinking! Tim! She's drinking!'

I laugh out loud, what a relief!

'She carefully drank a few sips this morning. And she also pulled off and ate some leaves from a branch.'

It warms my heart to hear the joy in his voice. That means there's hope again, while everyone had already given up. When I hang up the phone, I immediately call Marie to pour out my heart. My voice is cracking: 'Marieke, Mala is doing a little better. I wasn't expecting that anymore.' Marie is almost as happy as I am, because she has also known Mala for years.

On the fifth day, Mala starts eating well again and on day six she delights us with a dung ball.

It's clear that her teeth are the problem, so the only thing we can do is adjust her diet. An elephant would not be able to survive on pellets alone, as they also need roughage. We therefore also provide hay that has been pre-chopped by the grinder, so the strands are shorter and easier to chew.

Animals in captivity usually live longer than animals in the wild, so it makes sense that we should also adjust care and focus on a geriatric form of medicine.

Two years later, Mala is still healthy, as one of the oldest elephants in all of Europe.
In the wild, Mala would have eventually started looking for easily digestible food, simply because she could no longer chew properly. So most old elephants end up in a place with that kind of food, where they eventually die of old age. That's why there are legends of elephant graveyards, mysterious places where elephants die. But there's not much mystery to it if you know the explanation: they gather there because of the food and die there due to old age. But not Mala. Luckily, not Mala.

31. We are desperate

How do we get a gorilla into a CT scanner? That's the question we're all asking ourselves when it turns out that a CT scan may tell us more about Lomako, the gorilla in question. Lomako came to Pairi Daiza with his brother from Artis Zoo in Amsterdam a few years ago. He is still a subadult and therefore not yet a silverback. Lomako has been losing weight for a while, despite nutritional monitoring, so there is more going on here. An echocardiogram and abdominal ultrasound have already been performed, blood has been taken, and he has received symptomatic treatment with extra vitamins to counteract nutritional deficiencies. According to the results, everything was normal, apart from the blood values which indicated an excessive muscle breakdown. The weight loss could therefore be due to the loss of muscle, as a result of a primary muscle problem or an immunity issue.

'The opening of the scanner must be large enough,' I think aloud. 'At the animal clinic in Merelbeke, that's not the case. Neither in other hospitals. But... I know one place where it might just work.'

The place is a private animal clinic near Sint-Niklaas; I know one of the owners. So I immediately call him.

'Filip, can I come over with a gorilla?'

Filip initially laughs, because it's not a question he gets every day. On the contrary.

He quickly responds when he hears the story.

'Come over!'

I arrange transportation for Lomako through a transport company that only transports animals, and together with the keepers, I prepare him for his trip. Animal transports between zoos are almost a daily occurrence and it's important that it happens professionally. Some companies have therefore specialized in transporting wild animals. They have specially adapted trucks with climate control and cameras to observe the animals during the journey, and the crates they use have been designed specifically for each species, so that they can transport the animals safely and comfortably.

Lomako, just like the other gorillas, is trained to receive an injection by hand. Our keepers are extremely dedicated and experienced, and, above all, very patient. A few times a week they do a medical training with the gorillas. During this training, various medical procedures are simulated such as opening the mouth to examine the teeth, offering the back to listen to the lungs, offering the ear to measure the temperature, and also offering the upper arm to receive an injection. This is taught step by step and is solely based on positive reinforcement. That means that good behavior is rewarded. The animal participates on a voluntary basis and can stop whenever it wants. To teach these behaviors, the 'bridge reward' system is used. The 'bridge' is a signal, often a whistle, that indicates the exact point of the behavior the trainer wants to achieve. Immediately after the bridge, the animal receives a reward, something they enjoy, like a piece of apple or banana. The animal quickly makes the connection between the behavior, the bridge and the reward, and will therefore repeat this behavior to receive a reward. In the case of an injection by hand, the keeper asks for 'shoulder', after which the gorilla presents his shoulder. He can then administer the injection. The great advantage of this training is that a medical examination becomes a positive and stress-free experience for the animal, as well as for the veterinarian.

Once Lomako has had his shot and is out, we can move him. First, he's placed on a stretcher because Lomako, although he has lost weight, still weighs over 220 pounds. He's then laid into a specialized transport box for the journey so that we would still be safe should he wake up before we arrive at the clinic.

Together with Kevin, one of the keepers, I ride at the front. With Lomako in tow, we drive straight to the animal clinic where Filip is already waiting for us. So is Kathleen, an internal disease specialist and Filip's wife. I also asked her to be there to do a gastroscopy, to rule out a possible ulcer.

'Everything is ready,' says Filip when we greet him. He seems a bit nervous, which I can't blame him for. He has never had a gorilla in

his CT scanner before, but this is also new for us. I want to monitor Lomako closely, so he doesn't have to know anything about this and is as comfortable as possible.
The carrier opens the truck where Lomako is sitting. He seems to be asleep still. The crate is taken out of the truck with a forklift and driven to the CT scanner. 'Gorilla incoming,' Filip shouts, so everyone moves aside.
'Before I open the box, I first need to administer a new dose of ketamine,' I reassure everyone. I don't want to take any risks and the timing is good. Lomako will be out for a little while longer.
After the top-up injection, I carefully open the transport box and together we pull the gorilla out. Kevin stands behind Lomako and lifts him upright with his arms under his shoulders. This is the easiest way to intubate a gorilla, which Kevin of course knows because he has done this often enough with me. With two cords behind the canines, he pulls the head up and the mouth open. I'm now standing in front of Lomako and looking right into his mouth. I can see the larynx with the laryngoscope and insert the tube. I secure the tube with a cord behind Lomako's head so it can't move. Using the clinic's hoisting system that is normally used for horses, we eventually get Lomako onto the scanner table.
'Now it's your turn, Kathleen,' I say.
Kathleen takes the gastroscope in her hands and inserts it into the mouth. All the while, she looks at a monitor as she advances the scope further. She locates the esophagus and gently nudges the scope deeper. She carefully examines the wall to see if there is any damage. Little by little, she slides the scope further until it reaches the stomach. Here she conducts a thorough examination and then comes back up. 'Nothing abnormal found,' she says.
After this first examination, we position Lomako carefully on the CT scanner's table, then strap him in. I check the anesthesia one last time. 'He's ready,' I decide. 'Now it's our turn,' I add when I see everyone hesitating a bit.

Everyone seems to be overwhelmed. I am too. It's a bit surreal to see a gorilla lying there so defenseless. Kevin, me... We all know him as the tough guy, lively and playful.

Due to the weight loss, he has lost a lot of his charisma and now that he is lying here like this, it's quite a sad sight.
'Come on. We got this.'
'Everyone outside!' Filip calls out. 'We're starting the scan.' When the room is empty, Lomako is slid into the scanner with the push of a button. We watch behind the glass as images are formed on the computer screen. The interpretation of those images will have to wait a bit, as a human specialist in diagnostic imaging will still need to review them. Lomako is slid back out of the scanner. His outing is over.
'Well done everyone,' I say. 'Well done, Lomako.' I carry out a final check and gently stroke his head before he's loaded back into the box and we take him back to the zoo. Before we close the door of the box, he receives an injection to wake up again, so he can immediately be placed back in his enclosure as soon as we arrive. I'm trying not to show it to the keepers, but I'm very worried about his condition. We have been searching for several months now and still don't know what he has.
Lomako has weathered his trip well, but it's striking how much weaker he is compared to a few days ago. He is visibly deterioating and that worries everyone.
A few days later, Filip calls me.
'I have forwarded the images to a human specialist, and he sees a kind of fibrosis or scarring in the muscles. That can have various causes, including a genetic one. Maybe you should investigate further in that direction.'
'A genetic cause,' I think. 'What can be done about it? Can anything be done at all? And who can help with that?'
After an online search, I find the neuromuscular reference center at the University Hospital in Ghent. There, they conduct research into

muscle diseases. I put on my big boy pants and call the phone number on the website.

'Good morning, ma'am, I'm a veterinarian and have a problem with a gorilla. Could you help, please?'

The lady on the other end of the line is startled by my question, but tells me to write an email detailing the issue. She promises to forward that email to the relevant professors. No sooner said than done, and that same day I get call back.

'Hello colleague, it's Dr. Vanlander. I got your email, how can I help?'

I recount the whole story, and the doctor replies:

'That reminds me of central core disease, or CDC for short, a rare genetic muscle disease that occurs in 1 out of 1 million people. A muscle biopsy can clarify this.'

We agree to a muscle biopsy as soon as possible to see if we are finally on the right track. I hope so. I really hope so.

Now we have a possible diagnosis, but when I look up more about the disease, I don't exactly feel happy. The brochure I downloaded says the following: 'The general symptoms of CDC are muscle weakness and decreased muscle tone. CDC is caused by a mutation in the genetic material: in the RYR1gene of the DNA. The disease is usually inherited in an autosomal dominant manner. This means that a child can develop the disease if they inherit the abnormal gene from one of the parents. The parent usually has the disease themselves, possibly in a mild form. Each child of a parent with the disease has a 50% chance of getting the disease.'

I sigh. We also have Lomako's brother here; surely he won't be positive as well? That's my initial thought. I continue reading.

'The severity of the symptoms can vary greatly. Sometimes the symptoms are so limited that central core myopathy is only diagnosed in a parent when the disease manifests in the child.' I know Lomako's father is the breeding male in Amsterdam. So how many offspring are there already? I need to inform the EEPcoordinator of the gorillas if this is confirmed. But my first and most important task now is to inform the keepers, because they are heartbroken to see their gorilla suffering like this.

'We are distraught...' one of them confides in me after I share my suspicions with them. The six gorillas in the zoo have a team of three keepers. The keepers are very close to them, which is not surprising. Only elephants, marine mammals and great apes have their own dedicated keepers who solely take care of them. Other keepers still switch between different animal species. The gorilla team knows those six animals inside out. That's why I also believe it's important to discuss everything with them, to involve them in every step of the examinations. I don't want to damage their trust, and one way to avoid that is by communicating well.
'I understand,' I reply. 'The desperation you feel, well I just feel so helpless. But we are doing all we can, you have to remember that. Now we need to prepare for another anesthesia to do a muscle biopsy.'
A few days later, I receive a phone call from the same keeper.
'Lomako has passed away. We found him dead in his enclosure this morning.'
Words fall short. The despair and powerlessness suddenly turn into sadness.
'We reviewed the video footage... He fell asleep peacefully ... And did not wake up again.'
I am somewhat reassured that Lomako passed away in his sleep.
It is now up to me to perform an autopsy on him, which will allow us to investigate the entire disease process. After the muscle biopsy, confirmation follows: Lomako does indeed have CDC, the same genetic muscle disorder that also occurs in humans.
Now that this is 100% confirmed, I'm tasked with setting a whole system in motion and informing the EEPcoordinator so that further research can be done on Lomako's parents' family tree. Based on the family tree, it should be checked whether any young animals have died, and from now on it is recommended not to breed with descendants of that lineage, as the gene is passed on by the parents. So apparently Lomako's father, who is in the Amsterdam zoo, also had an episode at one point, although he did get through it. Some time later, Lomako's brother, who also resides in our zoo, shows the same symptoms, but much less severe. That proves that some can live with

the disease, others show no symptoms at all, and some die from it. It is somewhat reassuring for us that the diagnosis had never been made in gorillas before. We therefore could not have done anything else for Lomaka than what we had done: give him the best care and continue to search for the cause.

Lomako was eventually given a private cremation, and his ashes have received a special place in the park. This is out of respect for the public and the team of keepers, who have taken Lomako and the other gorillas to their hearts as the charismatic animals they are.

32. A world first: Spix's macaw part 2

'Hey Tim, Martin here... Can you come to Berlin? I would like to discuss something with you.'

I'm sat on a bed in a hotel in Skopje, North Macedonia. I have just finished checking an elephant enclosure here to see if some elephants could come to the zoo. I know Martin from my time in Qatar. He is the owner of the Association for the Conservation of Threatened Parrots, ACTP for short, and breeds, among others, Spix's macaws. The sheikh I worked for in Qatar recently passed away, and, in consultation with his children, it was decided that Martin would take over all the Spix's macaws to continue the sheikh's life's work, the breeding program of the Spix's macaw, in Berlin.

Without a second's hesitation, I say: 'I'm on my way.' At the airport, I book a ticket to Berlin instead of boarding the flight to Brussels. After my time in Qatar, I secretly came to love the Spix's macaws. It's such a special bird and such a beautiful project, so I'm curious about what Martin wants to propose to me.

Martin is already waiting for me at the exit and we give each other a warm hug.

'What's so urgent?' I ask as we drive to the breeding center in the car.

'As you know, I have adopted all the birds, including the Spix's macaw, from Qatar. Because it's dangerous to keep all birds in one place due to a possible disease outbreak, I would like to suggest that Paira Daiza takes over some birds to spread the risk. What do you think?'

Of course Martin knows what I think, otherwise he wouldn't have called me.

'I do have to discuss this first with the boss.'

After I hang up the phone to explain the story to my boss, I say: 'Okay, we'll do it.'

An agreement is signed between ACTP, Pairi Daiza, and the Brazilian government, and so initially four Spix's macaws are brought to Belgium. We quickly decide that a breeding program should also be set up at Pairi Daiza, and a brand-new breeding center is built where there is room for ten breeding pairs.

When I was still working in Qatar, the sheikh had bought a 57,000-acre piece of land which included the tree the last Spix's macaw was stolen from. Together with my local team, we started habitat reconstruction by removing the animals from the land and restoring the creek systems. New trees were also planted. Meanwhile, this project has been continued by the Brazilian government and ACTP. ACTP has also purchased additional land in the Caatinga in Brazil, and in collaboration with Pairi Daiza, a breeding-release center is being built for the final step in this challenging project.

On a freezing February day in 2020, Martin, my boss, and I board a private flight to Petrolina in Brazil. Some of the birds will breed there, while others are the first birds that, after having been extinct for twenty years, are being flown back to be released into the wild. The arrival is a true celebration, and the parrots are welcomed by the Brazilian Minister of Conservation. After a press conference, the birds are transported further by road to the newly built breeding and release center in the Caatinga.

In Curaçao, the hometown of the Spix's macaw, the people are completely ecstatic because their lost treasure is back home after twenty years. People are laughing, singing, drinking, and coming together to celebrate the return of the Spix's macaw. We have been invited by the local school; the students are wearing T-shirts emblazoned with 'the Spix is back home' and plays are being performed.

But now the hard work begins for Cromwell, who has meanwhile moved from Qatar to Brazil, and his team, to prepare the macaws for a life in the wild. The young Spix's, who have been selected, will be placed together in an aviary with Illiger's macaws. Those are parrots that still live in the habitat of the Spix's macaw in the Caatinga and serve as a kind of teacher. One big question is how Spix's respond to birds of prey and, in turn, how birds of prey will respond to Spix's. A Spix's macaw has no natural enemies in captivity and the birds of prey have not seen a blue parrot for twenty years. These are all things that need to be taken into account. By placing the Spix's with the Illiger's, they will learn things from the Illiger's, who are familiar with the dangers of the Caatinga. When Illiger's spot a bird of prey, they let out an alarm call and start flying around frantically. The Spix's observe and replicate this, learning to recognize and respond to danger. In the aviary, the parrots also eat local food from the wild, and when the Illiger's eat this food, the Spix's follow suit. So a kind of 'Spix's school' is being set up.

After two years, I am back in the Caatinga. Tomorrow, the first Spix's macaws will be released into the wild after a 22- year absence. This is, without a doubt, the biggest day in my professional career. I'm so incredibly nervous that I don't get a wink of sleep that night for fear of missing the bus to the release site. Upon arrival, after an hour's drive on unpaved bumpy roads, there is an excited atmosphere among the select group of attendees. There's a birdwatching tent set up about twenty meters from the large release aviary, with small viewing holes from which we can observe everything. The aviary is 80 feet high and at the very top there is a food platform with a door next to it. Outside, 3 feet farther, there is another food platform to attract the Spix's.

Cromwell arrives on his ATV, as he does every morning, to feed the Spix's. He walks inside and puts the food on the platform. Then he does the same on the platform outside.

'I'm opening the door,' he calls out.

Everyone holds their breath; you could hear a pin drop. Is a Spix's macaw going to fly out? After about ten minutes, the Illiger's respond; they have the instinct to go outside and curiously fly to that bowl of food. They keep hanging around the aviary and then wild Illiger's join them and fly around, but the Spix's... they stay safe inside. They're sitting on the feeding platform inside and looking outside through the open door, but they are far from making any attempt to fly through that opening. Until suddenly... one Spix's macaw flies out, from one feeding platform to another, almost by accident. It's a few feet to fly, no farther, but it's enough: the Spix's macaw is back in

the wild. Emotions run high, crying tears of relief, we embrace each other, Martin, Cromwell, and I. We are part of history. An extinct species is no longer extinct today. A little later, another Spix's macaw is exploring outside the aviary and now both of them fly around. Every day, the Spix's will be fed and the door will remain open, so they can always come back whenever they want. That's what we call a 'soft release', which is the method with the highest chance of success.
When we arrive the next day, we already hear the characteristic screeching of the Spix's macaw, and when we look up, Spix's macaws are flying around above our heads. It's unbelievable.
For twelve years I have been working on this project, from Qatar to here at this aviary in Brazil. In a way, it is my life's work, but at the same time I am just a link in the chain. Without the sheikh, ACTP, Martin's unwavering enthusiasm, and Cromwell who dedicated his life to those Spix's macaws, this would not have been possible. Never before has man succeeded in reintroducing a parrot that had gone extinct in the wild back into its natural habitat. And it is mainly thanks to their efforts that we have achieved a world first. Personally, I am especially grateful to have been a part of this, knowing that the artificial insemination I introduced so many years ago has played an important role in the ultimate survival of this species. I hope that I can go to the Caatinga with my family very soon, so they can also enjoy seeing the Spix's in the wild themselves, because they also helped by coming to Qatar.

2017-present (2023): Practice Belgium - consulting firm in Qatar

After working in Pairi Daiza for a couple of years, I decided to open my own little practice at home, for in my downtime. My role had evolved more and more over the years from mainly veterinarian to mainly zoological director, and I felt that I was starting to miss the real veterinary procedures. We also always try to work as hands-off as possible in a zoo, because every intervention, every anesthesia, carries a potential risk for the patient.

Marie and I agreed that the practice should remain primarily a hobby to keep me happy as a veterinarian, alternating with the demanding job at Pairi Daiza. So in good spirits, I set up a practice in the old office of our house and began receiving clients. It was great to speak with customers again and just treat animals, big and small, without any pressure. I could vaccinate and sterilize dogs and cats again, examine lame horses, and deliver lambs, while also treating special animal species such as birds, reptiles, deer, and so on.

As my experience grew, I also received more requests from other zoos, mainly outside Belgium, to help them with new species and come up with new enclosures; and I was also asked to perform difficult anesthesias or to treat elephants with herpes from Belgium to Germany to Thailand.

The request to take care of the pandas in Qatar came

at the right time. We had just reintroduced the Spix's macaw into the wild and I felt that my time at Pairi Daiza was complete. I had helped set up many new projects over the past few years and brought in many new animal species, and it was all becoming a bit repetitive. So I decided to take the plunge and move to Qatar.
I have not regretted this decision for a second and am happier today than ever before.

33. Deadly easy, easily dead

On the examination table in front of me sits a chicken, Ria. She is battered from head to toe, and looks like she has been tortured with some kind of instrument. She has deep wounds on her back, her feathers have been torn out in various places, and the wounds have also affected her muscles. Tortured, by the neighbor's dog to be precise.

'He walked in without us knowing,' Suzanne, the owner of the chicken, says, upset.

'Until Ria started cackling like crazy and a fight to the death broke out,' she explains.

Right now it does seem like the dog has won that fight, as the chicken seems to be barely hanging on by a thread.

'You have to save her,' Suzanne says. 'Ria is my favorite chicken. She just roams freely at home; she's so sweet and just comes to me when I call her name!'

A favorite chicken, but still just a chicken, I think. Though I don't say that out loud. If this animal means a lot to someone, I won't argue with that.

My rule is as follows: I provide the customer with all the information, and the customer does what they want with it. I always try to be honest, and I don't beat around the bush. Also, the financial considerations are not for me to make. You may wonder whether it's worth treating a chicken that costs 20 bucks for a few hundred dollars, but only the owner of that chicken can answer that. When people decide to go to the vet anyway, the animal often has an emotional value far greater than its financial value.

'If possible, I really want you to treat her. No matter the cost...'

'Then I'll treat her,' I say. A burden visibly lifts off Suzanne's shoulders. Ria seems to have her own thoughts about it.

As Suzanne leaves, I go to the living room, where my oldest son Jonah is sitting on the couch.

'There's work to be done,' I say cheerfully. He immediately knows what that means, and as he excitedly jumps up to assist me I don't mention that it involves a chicken.

'Oh,' is his reaction upon seeing the patient in distress. 'A chicken.'

'Ria.'

Jonah has become my regular assistant in the home practice over the years. He has always had a great interest in animals, especially birds, and he finds it fascinating to see me at work. Jonah rears special chicken breeds such as cochins and fighting chickens, and competes with pigeons in long-distance races. He also went to Brazil to check on the Spix's macaw project, and had the time of his life. Little by little, I am teaching him things he can help me with, especially the anesthesia of the animals that end up on my treatment table. Jef and Laura-Marie are less interested in my work. They do help when there's no other option, but they prefer to just pop in quickly to say hello and then leave.

In the case of Ria, Jonah will maintain the anesthesia and provide me with the necessary materials. The ultimate responsibility for anesthesia of course lies with me; that's something I don't delegate. I use gas anesthesia, which allows me to dose much more accurately and also work much longer with more control. Jonah holds Ria tight and I put a small mask on her nose. I set the oxygen to 34 ounces per minute and open the isoflurane gas to 5 volume percent. Jonah feels the chicken starting to relax in his hands after about thirty seconds, until it falls asleep completely. 'Just put her on the table, Jonah,' I say. 'We're going to intubate her.' Jonah immediately knows what is expected of him and opens her mouth so I can see the larynx. With a steady hand I slide a small tube into her windpipe and then I tape it to her beak so it can't accidentally slip out. Jonah immediately connects the tube to the breathing hose. 'Set the isoflurane to 2.5.' Jonah turns the container until the arrow indicates 2.5.

Birds have lungs, but also an air sac system that helps them to fly. In these air sacs, there is no gas exchange like in the lungs. However, during anesthesia, they can fill up with isoflurane, the anesthetic gas we use in birds. That causes extra gas to build up in the birds' bodies, which can lead to overdosing and, in the worst case scenario, death.

That makes the anesthesia of birds 'deadly easy,' but they are also 'easily dead'.

I start by disinfecting the wounds and assessing them.
'The spine has not been hit,' I say. 'Good news already. I can usually suture the bite wounds.'
'Well, it's something different than an elephant or a hippopotamus,' Jonah remarks sarcastically.
I laugh. It's true. And it's something I often hear in the practice. My work at the zoo is mainly 'hands-off,' which means that intervention should only happen when absolutely necessary. My work at the veterinary practice at home is mainly 'hands-on': sterilizing or neutering dogs and cats, treating different animal species, and interacting with customers, all of which I value greatly. The work at the practice also keeps me sharp. I'm a veterinarian who doesn't back down easily, thanks to my experience. Removing a large tumor from a small gecko, performing surgery on a hamster or neutering a rabbit... I do it all Unless it would not be in the best interest of the animal, then I will also be honest and recommend palliative care or euthanasia.
So whether it's an elephant, hippo, dog or chicken, I do it all with the same care, enthusiasm and passion.
Three hours later, I have used six boxes of sutures, which is about eight feet of suture material. For comparison, when sterilizing a cat, I only need one of those boxes.
'There, that's done,' I decide, seemingly relieving Jonah from some kind of suffering as well. It's eleven o'clock Saturday night, a time when a teenager might want to be doing something else.
'You did well again,' I compliment him. I'm not even lying, it's fantastic to see how much he's learning here and how eager to learn he usually is. Except maybe on a Saturday night. As a father, I beam with pride to see him so engaged, and in those moments I realize how lucky I am that we share that passion for animals together.
Ria will be hospitalized for tonight and can go back home the next

day. She still has a long and probably happy life ahead of her, but the attack by the dog has also affected her egg factory: Ria will never be able to lay eggs with shells anymore. Although at the end of the day, that is just minor stuff, after her life or death battle.

34. The freezer is full

The chicken we patched up last night had barely left the clinic when the phone in the practice starts ringing again. Something tells me there won't be any rolls or croissants for me this Sunday.

'We have two small hyenas in transit here at Brussels Airport; they're passing through from Africa to Portugal. We took a look at them, and one of them has diarrhea and shows signs of dehydration. We're not sure who to call, so maybe you could examine them for us?'

A phone call like this is always a surprise. The people of the FASFC, the Federal Agency for the Safety of the Food Chain, in collaboration with customs, inspect all live animals or products of animal origin entering the European Union. Hyenas passing through definitely fall into this category. If those hyenas are not completely healthy, they could pose a danger to public and animal health, which is why strict controls are necessary. And in this case also an examination.

'I can do that,' I reply. 'But the animals would have to come to the practice. They might need an IV or anesthesia, and I can't possibly bring all my equipment.'

'That can be arranged!'

No more than five minutes later, I receive another phone call.

'Jeff here, I just spoke with the FASFC. I'll handle the transit in Brussels and if it's convenient for you, I can come over now.'

We quickly make arrangements then I hang up the phone. I rush into the living room, while Marie and the children are sitting calmly around the table. There are even some rolls and croissants left.

'There's Hyena's on the way!' I call out excitedly.

Laura-Marie and Jef give me a confused look and Marie wonders out loud whether that's dangerous. The only one sharing my enthusiasm is Jonah.

'Can I help?' An unnecessary question.

A little later, the doorbell of the practice rings. Jeff, the man I spoke to earlier, is at the door. Next to him are two crates, each containing one hyena.

'Just give me a heads up when they need to be picked up again.'
Jonah and I are left with two hyenas on the porch. We move the crates inside and I immediately grab an electric screwdriver to open the doors. The crates are well secured for transportation. All crates must comply with the IATArules, the rules of the International Air Transport Association. They need to have a tray for feces, need to meet minimum dimensions and have an opening for food and water. Naturally, all crates must be securely closed so that no animals can go wandering about the airplane. For hyenas, this usually means there is a double door. The first one is a closed door made of wood or metal, and then there is another door with mesh or bars.
We then see the two little animals. I estimate that the hyenas are about twenty weeks old, but looking at their behavior, they seem to think they're adults. They hiss, growl, and puff their manes to appear larger. They are ready to attack.
'Um,' Jonah hesitates. 'How are you going to examine them?'
'Simple,' I say. 'By taking them out of those cages.'
Jonah looks at me questioningly, but I explain to him how we will proceed.
'We let them come out of the box one by one. As soon as they're out, we throw a cloth over their head and grab them by the neck. You hold them tight while I examine them.'
Jonah doesn't seem very reassured, but follows my instructions.
We start with the hyena that looks the worst. We place the cage on the floor and open the door. He slowly takes a few steps outside. I'm standing over the cage with a towel, and Jonah is standing behind me so he is still a bit protected. I do feel responsible for him and I really don't want to explain to Marie that Jonah was bitten by a hyena. As soon as the hyena is out, I throw a large towel over its body and head and grab it by the scruff of the neck through the towel. This doesn't take more than five seconds. 'Good, now you take over, Jonah.'
Jonah holds the animal firmly while I listen to its breathing and heart with the stethoscope. I also listen to the bowel sounds and the frequency has clearly increased. I feel the stomach and feel some gas. I immediately notice from the skin that the hyena is showing signs

of dehydration, as it lacks elasticity.
'Were going to treat symptomatically,' I explain. That means we will treat the diarrhea without knowing the cause, otherwise we would have to send samples to the lab, which is difficult on a Sunday. I start by administering fluid subcutaneously to combat the dehydration. The hyena also receives Buscopan for the spasmodic sounds I hear in the intestines, and I decide to administer some antibiotics as well. After the treatment, we push the animal back into the box.
'Next!' I say to Jonah, who is already in position to throw the cloth over the head of the other hyena.
This second specimen is in better shape. Administering fluid is sufficient and antibiotics are not necessary.
'Not too bad after all,' I conclude when both animals are back in their crates. 'Though the sick hyena will need to be treated again a few more times. That means they have to stay here and we have to feed them. I still need to come up with something for that.'
'My chickens!' Jonah calls out. 'The freezer is full of them!' He looks at me wide-eyed and suddenly I realize what he's talking about. Jonah has just completed a project in his final year of high school where he compared three groups of chickens. The first group received hobby feed, the second group received industrial feed, and the third group had to make do with a composite feed that was homemade and based on the other two feeds. The chickens were fed for a while and at the end they were slaughtered to be weighed for an evaluation. Which is why our freezer is full of chickens. Twenty-four chickens, to be precise. It was fantastic seeing Jonah at work on his research. Every day he weighed the feed, checked the chickens and cleaned the coops. In the end, he concluded which feed provided the best growth and the best feed conversion ratio. The homemade feed had the worst results, but both the hobby and industrial feed gave very good results and therefore also tasty chickens.
But perhaps more importantly, we can now use those chickens to feed two young, hungry hyenas and help them recover. After a few feedings and treatments, they are ready to travel again. And we have some more space in our freezer again.

35. It sounds easier than it is

'There's a pig on the loose in a forest here and we can't find anyone to help us catch it. Can you come over to shoot it with your tranquilizer? A new owner has been found who wants to take over the animal.'

With an apologetic look, I glance at my daughter Laura-Marie, who immediately knows what that means. Today should be a father-daughter day, a day when we spend some quality time together. Veterinary medicine doesn't mean much to her, but she's crazy about horses. A trip to Oostende Koerse to watch the horse races is the ideal outing for her.

'I want to,' I say quickly. 'But it's not easy to anesthetize a pig. A pig like that isn't put to sleep easily, and the products needed for anesthesia are expensive.'

'We'll take care of that,' they say.

'Fancy catching a pig with me?' I ask Laura-Marie after the phone call ends. 'If everything goes smoothly, we will definitely still be back in time to see the horse races.'

A little later, Laura-Marie and I arrive at the forest where the pig is said to be hiding.

'So many people,' Laura-Marie remarks.

There's indeed a group of about ten men gathered. Some are from the animal shelter, others from forest management, and others are random passersby who stop out of curiosity. The people from the animal shelter already have a large kennel ready to transport the pig.

'Here's the pig,' they say immediately. 'Come take a look. It was dumped by someone who wanted to get rid of it. Terrible when people do something like that.'

Laura-Marie and I are led through a path in the forest to the pig.

'What?' I say in surprise when I see it.

'Piglets!' Laura-Marie says excitedly.

The pig is lying stretched out on the ground, unfazed by our visit, with ten piglets greedily drinking at its belly. The piglets seem to be a few weeks old.

'Didn't we mention that?' the person I spoke to earlier on the phone asks a bit hesitantly, aware of what he had kept from me.

'No,' I sigh. 'You didn't mention that. Do you at least have a net to catch those piglets?'

'Uhm…'

I've heard enough; I'm on my own here. If I anesthetize the mother, we can first take the piglets and then her. I don't want to waste too much time, so I send someone to get a net and go back to the car with Laura-Marie to grab my gun and tranquilizers.

Everyone is dead quiet as I aim my gun at the pig, and remains silent until the pig falls asleep not long after the tranquilizer dart pierces her buttock. The piglets stay with the mother, as predicted. But that changes when they realize that their mother no longer responds to their presence.

'Oh no,' I say quietly.

One by one, the piglets walk away from the mother, eventually running off in a group. What follows looks like a kind of slapstick video: about ten adults run around like headless chickens trying to catch the piglets. Laura-Marie was smart enough to watch everything from a distance without getting her hands dirty. She still had to go to Oostende Koerse!

I quickly put the pig in the kennel, and after she wakes up she will attract the piglets with her grunting. Although it sounds easier than it is. Eventually, it took ten minutes to sedate and put the pig to sleep, but four hours to catch those ten piglets. We didn't make it to Oostende Koerse.

36. Mankind, animal kingdom

'Bruno! I haven't heard from you in a long time,' I say enthusiastically when an old friend is on the line.

'Tim, I have a question... A friend of mine, a football player who plays for the Red Devils, has moved from Tongeren to Liège. In Tongeren, he has some land where fallow deer roam. Would you be up for tranquilizing those deer to transport them to Liège?

'Yes of course, I would even enjoy that,' I say immediately. 'Just send me the coordinates.'

A few phone calls and days later, I drive to Tongeren on a Saturday, together with Laura-Marie. Upon arrival, we drive onto the beautiful courtyard of an old farm, but the deer are nowhere to be seen. We get out of the vehicle and are welcomed by a woman.

'We'll take a short walk to the deer,' she says. 'I'm Rachel, by the way.'

Laura-Marie and I follow her through an old monumental arch to the other side and arrive at a parking lot. After we have crossed the parking lot, we arrive at the place where the deer live.

'This is where the plot of land starts,' says Rachel.

Laura-Marie and I look at each other.

'Dad…' she says quietly. 'It's really big here. And there is no meadow here?'

I shrug my shoulders warily and signal that we better follow Rachel. She leads us through a stretch of forest to eventually arrive at a large meadow: but still there is not a single deer to be seen.

'They must be around here somewhere,' Rachel says, but I notice she is looking around doubtfully.

Laura-Marie and I continue walking when suddenly a dozen deer dart out of the tall grass just a few feet away from us. They set off running at lightning speed. Immediately after that, we see even more deer appear. We can count about twenty of them, but they stay at a safe distance of about 150 feet.

'Ah, there they are,' says Rachel, pointing to the deer. 'See? Well, can you catch them now?'
I look at Laura-Marie and we can barely suppress a smile.
'Well, Rachel,' I say delicately. 'I'm afraid it won't be so simple. This piece of land is several acres, the deer roam freely and can flee into the forest to hide. They don't come closer than 150 feet, which is too far to shoot them with the tranquilizer gun. I'm afraid this will take some time. I'll make a plan and come back later.'
When Laura-Marie and I drive away, we start chatting animatedly about our deer experience.
'How are you going to do that, dad?'
'Well hun, the only way to try this is by building 'bomas'. Those are corral traps built in the wild in Africa for gazelles and antelopes. Animals can be fed there and when they are in the boma, the door is closed so they can be captured in a smaller area.'
'Oh, yeah,' Laura-Marie says, a little impressed. 'That sounds like a good idea.'
I think so too, but where on earth do I find a boma in Belgium?
Once home, I immediately search the Internet for where I can buy bomas in Europe. There are many deer farms in England, so I might be able to find something there. But unfortunately, I can't find any suitable material that is light enough to build with in a forest. Finally, I end up at Heras fences, a company well known to us. I see that they have lots of options, and find some fences that seem suitable if I can cover them with the included black plastic covers, so the deer can't see through them.
I prepare the quote for my client including the installation of these fences, the anesthesia and the transportation of the deer to their new home. I'm happy when the customer says I can start. To be honest, I'm still not sure if this will succeed, but my desire is greater than the fear of failure.
'Jonah! Jef,' I call. 'Come downstairs!'
The boys are probably scared that they are in trouble, so I immediately explain why I need them.
'Tomorrow the fencing will be delivered in Tongeren and I need your

help to set up the boma for the deer. That's heavy work, so I can't do it alone.'

After some muttering and grumbling from my sons, I manage to convince them to come help me. Jef and Jonah actually think it's pretty cool that it's at a famous soccer player's home.

The next day the three of us are in the car on our way to Tongeren.

'Boys, here's the plan. That's how we're going to build the boma. Take a good look. The entrance is located front right, and the deer go through a narrow corridor into the first enclosure at the back right corner. Then we build a second enclosure with the entrance at the front again so that the deer have to zigzag through the boma, making them go deeper into it and come out less quickly.

'Why would the deer want to go in there?' Jonah wonders out loud. 'Isn't that a foreign object in their environment?'

A valid point. That's why I asked Rachel in advance to feed the deer each day, for a few weeks to a month. First, the feed is placed at the entrance and then, when we see it disappear, we place it deeper and deeper into the boma, until it is all the way at the back of the second enclosure. Rachel will have to check if the deer come more often, for example, in the morning or evening, so we know when the gate should be closed and when I should come to administer the anesthesia.

When we arrive in Tongeren, we get straight to work. It's a beautiful summery day in October so we can enjoy the sunshine as we work. Jonah and Jef are becoming real bears, sweat dripping from their faces as they walk around erecting the fences. I take my role of delegating seriously and make sure they work safely. Gradually, the boma takes shape, and the boys start to see that the plan might actually work. Something they had doubts about. We hang the black plastic sheets on the fences and reinforce them with extra metal pins on the outside, so the deer can't knock them over if they were to push against them. Once we are convinced that the structure is strong enough, we drive back home tired but satisfied after four hours of work.

'Now Rachel's work begins,' I say on the way. 'Hopefully she'll succeed in attracting the deer.'

After two weeks, I call Rachel to ask if the deer are already coming to eat.
'No, not yet,' she tells me. 'But they are getting close to the boma. The first week, they didn't even come within 300 feet of the thing, but now they're already sniffing at the fences and standing at the entrance. I'll keep at it.'
Two weeks later, I speak to Rachel again.
'Tim,' she sounds rushed. 'I've just arrived here, and there's lots of deer in the boma. I closed the door straightaway. Can you come now?'
I actually have other plans, but if we let those deer go now, they may never come back. So I change my plans and leave. Today is a school day, so I'm on my own. No sons or daughter to help.
Upon arrival, I can already hear the deer banging against the fence. 'It seems strong enough,' I mutter, more to myself than to Rachel. I carefully walk towards the boma as quietly as possible and quickly count the deer: fifteen in total, mostly females and their young. I concentrate as I prepare fifteen anesthesia darts in the car. First I test all the darts and needles to make sure they work, and then put the medetomidine in all the darts. Afterwards, I fill all the syringes with ketamine and attach the needles, pushing them firmly so they don't fall off. With my hand full of darts, I walk towards the boma. I press my first dart, insert it into my gun and stick the barrel through an opening between the fences. I aim, shoot, and.... Got it!
The first dart ends up in the buttock muscle of a deer. I repeat this procedure and shoot number 2, 3, 4 and 5. I go back to the car to get some more darts.
When my gun is loaded for number 6, I wait a moment, as I don't immediately recognize the deer, until number 1 lies down, 2 as well, 3, 4 and 5 start to stagger and eventually lie down too. Now I can continue. After fifteen shots, all the deer are asleep. Some are sleeping so deeply I can even hear them snore.
It's a strange sight when we walk in. Spread out over the entire boma are sleeping deer, some still with the dart in their neck or buttocks. All the deer must be lifted and carried to the horse trailer to be

placed neatly next to each other under anesthesia. All the animals are checked and receive a deworming shot, and then we head off to their new home, an hour's drive away, to a beautiful large farm in the Ardennes. Tired but satisfied, I drive home that evening. Our plan has been successful so far, but we have only caught half of the deer.

Ten days later, Rachel calls me again. When I see her number, I get excited because I expect she has caught deer again.

'The deer are no longer coming near the boma, not even within 600 feet. They avoid it like the plague.'

Disappointed, I hang up. What now? Plan B?

Marie and I are driving back to Tongeren. We have been married for eighteen years today, and I guess there can't be any better way to celebrate that than to go deer hunting together. Meanwhile, the new owners are already living in the house and they really want the deer to go away, because their children ride horses just like ours do. They would like to build a paddock, so we understand. Today we want to drive the deer to an open spot where I will be hiding ready to shoot them with my tranquilizer gun. We start in good spirits. We have gathered ten men to drive the deer, and I position myself in my hiding place.

The entire plan is unsuccessful. We have been walking around all day, but the deer are just smarter than us.

'Yeah Timmy, it's MAN-kind against the animal KING-dom, isn't it?' Marie remarks sarcastically.

Luckily, Bart, the new owner, did provide a Limburgian smurf tart to celebrate our wedding anniversary just a little. During my third piece of tart, we come up with plan C. Since that first time, the deer no longer come to the boma, but sit on the other side in the open meadow. Maybe we should set up the boma there.

We dismantle the structure and reposition it on the other side in the open meadow. We change the shape of the boma to a long narrow boma with one entrance then head back home; but not without agreeing on a new date in the very near future.

Once again I'm on my way to Tongeren, this time with Jonah and Jef, for what hopefully will be the last deer trapping. We are warmly welcomed by Bart and his team of helpers. Bart drives to the farm with the car and the deer are already looking up; they know this car means food. Bart places all the food deep in the boma, and then leaves. The deer come hesitantly and enter the structure. After a few minutes, we return in our cars and close the gate. This time we have them all. Most of them are big males with beautiful large antlers. And here I go again: making darts, taking my gun, loading a dart, shooting... A hit... One after the other, until they have all been sedated. Then we load the deer onto an open trailer. Jonah and Jef are allowed to sit alongside them and hold their antlers, then off we go to the horse trailer to load the deer. After an hour and a half and a warm goodbye from Bart and his family, the three of us drive to the Ardennes to release the last of the deer.

I call Marie. 'Hey sweetheart, humans are the animal royalty after all. It worked.'

I am extremely satisfied, because this is one of the most enjoyable things I have ever done in the field of veterinary medicine, even though they are just deer. The challenge was so great and the problem so complex, but we succeeded. And this time I didn't have to do it alone, as I had my family for support. My family, which, with Marie at the forefront, has always supported me in everything I did and do. Without them, I would never have been able to do what I do now and I am eternally grateful to them. They are the real heroes behind every story.

37. More pandas

'I work for an aquarium technology company and we are currently working on building a panda enclosure at the government zoo in Qatar.'

I raise my eyebrows as I read the first sentence of the email I just received. More pandas! I've been hearing about this for a while now. The enclosure should even be ready before the World Cup takes place in Qatar.

Curious, I read on.

'Our company applied to carry out the construction, but was not selected. The party that was chosen, however, has enlisted our help in building the actual enclosures. I heard through the grapevine that you are a specialist in pandas, hence my question: would you be willing and able to help in this project?'

Without wanting to immediately exclude or confirm anything, I reply to the email, asking: 'What would my task entail exactly?'

After some back-and-forth emailing, it becomes clear. So I agree. My job mainly consists of providing consultancy from Belgium, using my expertise to help them set up the enclosures and backstage of the new panda compound in Al Khor, Qatar. Because, currently, they have no such expertise there at all. The construction was carried out without any knowledge of the animals and their needs, there are no doors where doors should be, there are no drainage gutters for the water, there are too few enclosures, you name it. The project lasts fifteen months and I eventually manage to design and set up that enclosure completely as it should be, in collaboration with the Chinese specialists.

By the end of my assignment, I receive a new email.

'We notice our customer is still stuck on operational questions. They don't know where to import the right bamboo from, where to recruit veterinarians and keepers, and so on. They trust you and our company since after the first project. Would you be interested in coming to

lead the panda project here?'
I stare at my computer screen. The offer does interest me, especially since I am getting a bit tired of my current job. But I don't feel like moving to Qatar again. Not without my family, and actually not with my family either, because their whole life is in Belgium now.
'I would love to,' I reply. 'As long as this task can also be done remotely.'
Of course, it's not possible to take care of the pandas remotely, but in the end we come to a compromise: I will work full-time in Qatar for six months, and then switch to a flexible arrangement where I can return to Belgium regularly.
I immediately spring into action. I move to Doha and assemble a good team around me. The great advantage I have is that I worked in Qatar for a long time and therefore know good keepers whom I trust and vice versa. At the same time, coincidence brings me to Cissy, a Chinese-Canadian panda keeper who has gained a lot of knowledge about pandas in Hong Kong and Canada, who now also wants to join the team. I also find a veterinarian who can work full time.
The only thing missing now are the pandas themselves.
The biggest logistical challenge is the import of the bamboo. The diet of pandas consists of 95percent bamboo, which does not grow naturally in the desert, just like nothing else grows here. Once this is sorted out through suppliers in China and Europe, the transportation for the pandas can be arranged. To ensure their move goes smoothly, I first schedule a meeting with the government and the group of Chinese people who will lend out the pandas. Fortunately, those are people I know from the panda move to Belgium, which already takes away a lot of stress and offers reassurance to them and myself. We know that we will do everything to ensure the arrival and stay of the pandas goes smoothly. At that time, China is still in the midst of the Covid pandemic, which somewhat complicates the arrival. China is in lockdown, so the usual leaving party with attendees from both countries cannot be organized. So it's up to us to organize the arrival party, but it's actually too hot in Qatar this time of year to do that. The party will therefore not be held at the airport, but in the

Panda House itself, with the intention of sparing the pandas as much as possible.

The day the pandas are picked up in China, I'm on the plane with them. It's a strange flight, because we are not allowed to enter China. So we're flying from Doha to Bangkok, where two other crews will board to continue flying to Cheng Du. Even before the flight, I realize that this will be a very different experience from when I visited the pandas in Belgium. And I'm not wrong. Instead of being warmly welcomed everywhere, I have to wear a kind of white spacesuit, have a thermometer placed against my forehead everywhere I go, and everyone seems a little scared.

Upon arrival in Cheng Du, I see the panda boxes ready to go. They are loaded onto the plane using a *high loader*, followed by Mr. Dong and Dr. Wu, keeper and veterinarian. The first one I still remember from my time panda training in China, so after we're allowed to take off our protective clothing, we warmly greet each other.

'Congratulations,' he says. 'You are officially the only person who has ever picked up two pandas for two different zoos.'

It will be a cozy gathering, with only eight people on the plane.

'What cargo are we transporting?' the co-pilot asks me.

I laugh.

'You're doing a panda flight,' I explain.

The poor man's expression changes immediately and he becomes nervous.

'Pandas?' he asks, concerned.

'Pandas,' I laugh. 'Wait, I have something for you.'

I rummage around in the hold for a bit and then come back with some panda plush toys, a highly appreciated gift.

By morning, we arrive in Doha, where we are greeted by the press as is customary. The pilots happily wave their panda plush toys, my colleagues and I shake hands with the dignitaries, and the pandas are moved to a cooled truck to be taken to their enclosure.

From the airport, we drive under police escort to Al Khor, where a crowd is waiting for us. Pandamania is not just reserved for Belgium. The Belgian audience, however, is slightly less enthusiastic than the

Qataris, who need to be occasionally restrained. The crates containing the pandas are unloaded with a forklift to then be taken to their enclosure. First the male is released, then the female follows.
When I'm sure they're okay, I give a thumbs up: the arrival party can start. There is an original sword dance with Qatari children, a speech by the ambassador of China, and a speech by the director of the panda enclosure; it's quite an experience. I feel completely different during that ceremony than the first time I experienced such an event. In Belgium, I was more nervous, more anxious that something would go wrong. But after ten years of panda experience and well-maintained contacts in China that is clearly different now. I trust them, they trust me. And that's still the case now.
My assignment is still ongoing and this project is the cherry on top when it comes to my story with the pandas. The pandas have brought me so much knowledge and joy.
The next challenge is setting up a breeding program that can hopefully start soon. I closely monitor the pandas' health and I am ultimately responsible for the entire program. If something is wrong or a panda gets sick, then I have to solve it. And I do it with pleasure.

Live now, not tomorrow

I'm sitting at my desk in Qatar. The pandas are busy in the background. Si Hai is sleeping in a tree and Jing Jing is sitting on his bamboo platform eating. I look at them and can't shake the thought that pandas are a very important part of my professional career. Ten years ago, I left Qatar to come take care of pandas in Belgium, and now I have left Belgium to take care of pandas in Qatar: the circle of life!

The panda is definitely not my favorite animal, because it sleeps almost the entire day, but it is an animal that has a certain charisma and cuddliness and that brings people closer together. If I think more deeply about this, that's actually the essence of my job: connecting with people and bringing them closer together, all through and with animals.

Pandas, as well as Spix's macaws and elephants, are animals that have personally touched me and that touch a lot of people around me. These animals, individually or in a group, tell a story full of wisdom and connection.

Pandas have taught me a lot. First and foremost, they are incredibly interesting animals from a veterinary perspective. The heat cycle lasting 24 hours and the delayed implantation of the embryo, along with the challenge of confirming the pregnancy, makes it all very fascinating. But more than that, it's an animal with diplomatic significance, symbolizing friendship between two countries. Through the pandas I got to know a new culture, the Chinese culture, and came to love it. I have made friends on the other side of the world with the same interests, who make me feel at home every time I travel there. The panda is also black and white, which, in Chinese culture, symbolizes the balance that every person hopes to find within themselves: yin and yang. I think every person is looking for that a little bit, I know I do.

The Spix's macaw, a bird and therefore an animal that, as a true mammal guy, I never thought would touch me, has above all taught me this: unknown is unloved. As I delved deeper into the story in Qatar, Belgium, and Brazil, I grew to love this bird more and more. Similar to the panda, this is also a political bird, as different countries collaborate on this. And here I have made new friendships that are intense, beautiful, and lasting. Helping to save a species from extinction is a very humbling experience. It makes you reflect on what we, as humans, as a species and top predator, do to those other animal species around us and their habitat. We are expanding, without taking into account other, more vulnerable animal species. According to researchers, 100 animal species disappear every day and 28 percent of all animal and plant species are currently threatened. It's high time we all try, individually, to contribute something so that our children and grandchildren still have a world to live in.

The elephant, my great love. A magical animal, a gentle animal, an intelligent animal. My fondest moments as a zoo veterinarian are with the elephant. Seeing an elephant calf being born remains special. Every time again. The way the group receives and takes care of this little miracle can teach us so much as humans. Elephants live in a close-knit family society, doing everything together as a group. They are very aware that a chain is only as strong as its weakest link. In our increasingly individualistic society, we sometimes forget the people we love the most and become more and more selfish. We are caught in the rat race of working, working, and working some more. I have also been guilty of this myself, until a serious accident made me realize that living to work is completely wrong. From now on, I work to live, and for the rest, I mainly want to be happy with my family and the people I love.

The new balance in my life between work and family, yin and yang, I now guard with my life, like the elephant and the panda.

What the future holds, no one knows. And that might just be a good thing. If I am asked what I will do tomorrow or next year, I'm glad I don't know. If there's one thing I've learned from all those years of working with animals, it's to live in the 'now'. Every animal, small or large, goes about its business and follows its instinct to live, to survive. I wish that for everyone: live and enjoy now, not tomorrow.

Acknowledgments

I have to admit that writing this book has had a big impact on me. It has made me reflect on an important period in my life, both professionally and personally, and all the people who have walked part of their lives with me.

As a child, I was given all the opportunities by my parents to grow and study. Thanks to their support, I was able to become a veterinarian. The mouth speaks what the heart is full of. And she has been mentioned many times in different chapters, my rock, my support, my refuge: Marie. I only now realize, by writing this book, how much she has sacrificed by following me, but always with an open mind to make the best of it together. She is the strongest person I know and without her, I wouldn't have a career, let alone a book. So this book is also her book, my story is her story. Marieke, thank you for everything.

My children, Jonah, Jef, and Laura-Marie, all three wonderful people and yet so different. I hope that our adventures together will make you stronger and even more beautiful people. I know you didn't have a choice and had to come along, but I've seen you grow everywhere into the beautiful young adults you are. Stay true to yourselves, that's perfect.

The person who shaped me as a veterinarian is Jaak. He took me by the hand as a young veterinarian and taught me the basics, but above all: he gave and still gives me unconditional friendship.

I certainly cannot forget the many colleagues over the years, especially the animal keepers, I have had the pleasure of working with. I have learned so much from your passion. You are the cornerstone of every zoo, and I am glad that you let me into your world.

And you, readers, thank you for buying and reading this book. I hope you enjoyed it.

I, for one, have enjoyed writing it for you.

Thank you

www.lannoo.com
Register on our website and we will regularly send you a newsletter with information about new books and interesting, exclusive offers.

EDITORIAL Nele Reymen, Mike Newton
PHOTOGRAPHY COVER: Noortje Palmers
DESIGN: Studio Vonk & De Boer

If you have any comments or questions, please contact our editorial team:
redactielifestyle@lannoo.com

D/2025/45/453
ISBN: 9789059960633